DATE DUE

ADVANCES IN NEUROLOGY
Volume 18

Advances in Neurology

INTERNATIONAL ADVISORY BOARD

Advances in Neurology
Volume 18

Hemi-Inattention
and
Hemisphere Specialization

Edited by

Edwin A. Weinstein, M.D.

Professor of Neurology
Mount Sinai School of Medicine and
Chief of Neurology
Veterans Administration Hospital
Bronx, New York

Robert P. Friedland, M.D.

Department of Neurology
Mount Sinai School of Medicine
of The City University of New York
New York, New York

Raven Press ▪ New York

Raven Press, 1140 Avenue of the Americas, New York, New York 10036

Library of Congress Cataloging in Publication Data

Main entry under title:

Hemi-inattention and hemisphere specialization.

    (Advances in neurology; v. 18)
    Includes bibliographical references and index.
    1. Brain—Diseases. 2. Cerebral dominance.
3. Brain—Localization of functions. 4. Depersonaliza-
tion. I. Weinstein, Edwin A., 1909-   II. Friedland,
Robert P. III. Series. [DNLM: 1. Dominance,
Cerebral. W1 AD684H v. 18 / WL335 H488]
RC321.A276 vol. 18 [RC386.2] 616.8'08s [616.8]
ISBN 0–89004–115–6   77–5278

Preface

One of the most striking demonstrations that the cerebral hemispheres, though separate, are not equal is the phenomenon of hemi-inattention in which a person ignores, forgets about, disowns, or turns away from one side of the body and/or ambient space. Hemi-inattention, or hemi-neglect, occurs predominantly in association with lesions of the minor, right hemisphere. For years it has attracted the especial attention of neurologists who needed a respite from the intricacies of aphasia localization and classification, and wondered how the other half of the brain lived. The manifestations of hemi-inattention have also excited the imagination of those who marveled that one could exist in a demi-world where laterality determined reality.

Our efforts to understand hemi-inattention have paralleled the development of neurological concepts of deafferentation, of the body image, of perceptual interaction and rivalry, and of the activating mechanisms of the limbic reticular system. They have involved studies of vision and other discrete sensory systems, oculomotor mechanisms, memory, emotion, and language.

This volume is timely because of the rapid development of new methods of studying hemispheric laterality, specialization, balance, and inhibition. It is an attempt to collate and compare the clinical findings of brain disease, psychophysiological measurements of attentional processes, the results of animal experimentation, and the effects of section of the corpus callosum, all of which have yielded data relevant to hemi-neglect.

Edwin A. Weinstein
Robert P. Friedland

Acknowledgments

We are indebted to the Veterans Administration, and in particular to Dr. Julius Wolf, Chief of Staff at the Bronx Veterans Administration Hospital, for his support. We would like to mention the support of PHS Grant #5 TOINS-05072 (Friedland), and Grant #05084 NINCOS, N.I.H., and the Waasdorp Fund for Stroke Research (Joynt). We would also like to express our appreciation to Mr. Ray Sawyer for his recording, and to Miss Sharon J. Quinn for her decoding and transcribing of many of the papers.

Advances in Neurology Series

Contents

Contributors

Morris B. Bender, M.D.
Department of Neurology
Mount Sinai School of Medicine
Fifth Avenue and 100th Street
New York, New York 10029

Robert Cohn, M.D.
Department of Neurology
Howard University College of Medicine
2400 Sixth Street
Washington, D.C. 20059

Leonard Diller, Ph.D.
Chief, Behavioral Science
Institute of Rehabilitation Medicine
New York University Medical Center
400 East 34th Street
New York, New York 10016

Robert P. Friedland, M.D.
Department of Neurology
Mount Sinai School of Medicine
Fifth Avenue and 100th Street
New York, New York 10029

Kenneth M. Heilman, M.D.
Department of Neurology
College of Medicine
University of Florida and
Veterans Administration Hospital
Gainesville, Florida 32610

Robert J. Joynt, M.D.
Department of Neurology
University of Rochester Medical Center
Rochester, New York 14642

Marcel Kinsbourne, M.D.
Neuropsychology Research Unit
The Hospital for Sick Children
555 University Avenue
Toronto, Ontario, Canada M5G 1X8

Jerre Levy, Ph.D.
Department of Psychology
University of Pennsylvania
3813 Walnut Street T3
Philadelphia, Pennsylvania 19174

Pedro Pasik, M.D.
Department of Neurology
Mount Sinai School of Medicine
Fifth Avenue and 100th Street
New York, New York 10029

Tauba Pasik, M.D.
Department of Neurology
Mount Sinai School of Medicine
Fifth Avenue and 100th Street
New York, New York 10029

Robert T. Watson, M.D.
Department of Neurology
College of Medicine
University of Florida and
Veterans Administration Hospital
Gainesville, Florida 32610

Joseph P. Weinberg
Institute of Rehabilitation Medicine
New York University Medical Center
400 East 34th Street
New York, New York 10016

Edwin A. Weinstein, M.D.
Department of Neurology
Mount Sinai School of Medicine and
Chief of Neurology
Veterans Administration Hospital
Bronx, New York 10468

Advances in Neurology, Vol. 18, edited by E. A. Weinstein and R. P. Friedland. Raven Press, New York © 1977.

Hemi-Inattention and Hemisphere Specialization: Introduction and Historical Review

Robert P. Friedland and Edwin A. Weinstein

Department of Neurology, Mount Sinai Medical School, New York, New York 10029; and Veterans Administration Hospital, Bronx, New York 10468

> . . . how false (is) a notion of experience that . . . would make it tantamount to the mere presence to the senses of an outward order. Millions of items of the outward order are present to my senses which never properly enter into my experience. Why? Because they have no *interest* for me. *My experience is what I agree to attend to.* Only those items which I *notice* shape my mind—without selective interest, experience is an utter chaos. Interest alone gives accent and emphasis, light and shade, background and foreground—intelligible perspective, in a word. It varies in every creature, but without it, the consciousness of every creature would be a gray chaotic indiscriminativeness, impossible for us even to conceive.
>
> *William James*
> *Principles of Psychology*
> *1890*

One hundred years ago, in 1876, John Hughlings Jackson described a case of "imperception," which contained many of the features of the condition that we will take up today (66). The patient, in reading, began at the lower right corner and tried to read backward. When asked if it was because she could not see, the patient replied, "No, *she* didn't think it was. *She* didn't seem to know how." She did not know places, persons, and objects, calling a penny a "sovereign" and the strings of a nurse's cap "long tails." She was sometimes withdrawn and unresponsive, and at other times showed no mental imperfection of consequence. In response to the argument that she was mentally confused, Jackson replied that if she was, she was confused only for objects, persons, and places. She also had difficulty in dressing and finding her way about the streets. The patient developed a left hemiplegia. A hemianopia could not be demonstrated, as it was impossible for her to keep her gaze fixed on a central point. At autopsy, a glioma of the right posterior (temporal) lobe was found by Sir William Gowers. In modern terminology, the patient would be said to have left visual hemi-inattention, disorientation for place and person, nonaphasic misnaming, dressing apraxia, topographical disorientation, and motor impersistence.

Since Jackson's time, there have been many case reports of hemi-inattention or hemi-neglect. New methods of observation have been introduced; animal models have been made and various theories offered. Although our knowledge of hemisphere specialization has advanced, certain problems relevant to the understanding of hemi-inattention remain. These are the definition of hemi-inattention itself, the relationship of extinction to the other manifestations of hemi-neglect, the relationships to other aspects of altered behavior, and the predominance of right-hemisphere over left-hemisphere lesions. In this introduction, we will review the phenomenological, historical, experimental, and theoretical perspectives in order to present the essential background of the papers that follow.

PHENOMENOLOGY

Patients with hemi-inattention may fail to recognize the limbs on one side of the body as their own. They may attend to events and notice people only on one side or respond only when addressed from one side. In drawing a figure, they may omit, distort, or misplace parts of an arm and/or leg, or an eye or ear on one side. Details may be missing from one half of a drawing of a house, flower, tree, or clock. In reading, the patient leaves out words and letters on one side, or notices only one side of an open book. The hemi-inattentive patient may fail to pick up coins on one side when presented with a horizontal or semicircular arrangement. A line may be bisected asymmetrically.

Hemi-inattentive patients may deviate their head and eyes constantly to the good side and may fail to look to the affected side on command or in pursuit. Macdonald Critchley (27) describes the behavior of patients who, when asked to raise their arms, elevate only the extremity on the "attentive" side. Similarly, when the patient is asked to grasp his ears, he may do so only with his unaffected hand, groping in space or grasping his cheek or hair with the affected hand. The patient may neglect to wear one sleeve or slipper, forget to place one foot on the rest of a wheelchair, or neglect to lock or unlock a wheelchair on one side. Hemi-inattentive subjects have been noticed to eat from only one side of a tray and to shave completely only one half of the face. A recent case report described the behavior of a chess player who ignored the pieces on one side of the board. Critchley (27) reported the case of an orchestra conductor who ignored the musicians on one side of the stage. Unilateral autotopagnosia may be seen, with inability to point to or name body parts only on one side.

It was recognized early that the essential feature of these phenomena is that they are not accountable solely in terms of sensory or motor deficit. Patients with only dense homonymous or bitemporal hemianopias may exhibit no evidence of visual hemi-neglect, and are generally able to draw and read without any asymmetry in their performance. Patients with even severe hemisensory deficit or hemiparesis may also show no evidence of hemi-inattention and may remain well aware of the presence and disability of the affected extremities. As pointed out by Battersby et al. (9), unilateral visual difficulties may not correspond to the specific areas of deficit found on perimetry. "There is not a localized area of spatial malfunction in other words, but rather a gradient of performance from the 'spared' to the impaired halves of space."

Failure of the patient to look to the affected side or raise the involved arm is likewise not due to the motor deficit per se. Full extraocular movements may be demonstrated on caloric stimulation, with passive head turning during fixation in patients whose head and eyes are deviated away from the impaired side. Subjects who do not raise both arms on command may be shown to have good power in other situations. There seems to be a reluctance rather than an inability.

Hemi-inattention occurs not only in the visual sphere, but may involve other sensory and motor functions as well. Cases are seen in which there is a loss of responsiveness to multiple stimuli from one side, including deficits in olfaction in one nostril, taste on one side of the tongue, and touch and vibration involving an entire half of the body. Such findings may be mistaken for hysterical, nonorganic sensory defects. Hemi-inattention may also be exhibited in the spheres of memory and emotion. Patients seem to forget about the limbs on one side, as in a case reported by Stanley Cobb (21). A most remarkable instance in our experience was that of an elderly lawyer who, when examined from his good side, behaved like the courtly, Southern gentleman that he was. When approached from his left side, however, he would make remarks like, "When are you going to get this over with you head shrinking son of a bitch?" Other examples of the emotional features of hemi-inattention include a patient with a left hemiplegia, reported by Zingerle in 1913 (157), who had erotic feelings in his "absent" left limbs, which he believed were those of a woman. Head and Holmes (54) told of a patient who was unable to go to his church "because he could not stand the hymns on his affected side," and who rubbed his hand constantly during the singing. They do not note whether the patient had neglect of the involved extremity. It appears that the profusion and diversity of the signs of hemi-neglect are limited only by the imagination of the patient and the attentiveness of the examiner.

Almost all authors agree that there is a predominance of right-hemisphere over left-hemisphere lesions in the occurrence of the forms of hemi-neglect that have been described. As will be considered later, these vary according to the method of study and criteria used. Hecaen, in a series of 59 cases, reported 51 patients with right, four with left, and four with bilateral hemisphere lesions (55,56). Weinstein and Cole (140) reported a right-hemisphere predominance of 22 to 3. Cohn (22), using asymmetry of figure drawing as the index, found a proportion of 3 to 1. Most recently Zarit and Kahn (156) report a ratio of 2 to 1. Battersby, Bender, Pollack, and Kahn (9) also found a greater incidence of right-hemisphere lesions but did not regard the difference as statistically significant.

Hemi-inattentive patients often appear unaware of their deficits. Even though an asymmetry is repeatedly brought to the patient's notice, he persists in his omissions and other errors. Patients verbally deny and minimize defects, or rationalize or confabulate about them. A woman with a left-sided neglect, when asked to count the people in the room, indicated only those on her right side. When asked about the others, she replied, "Oh, they don't count."

Hemi-inattention is most commonly seen with lesions of sudden onset, is most frequently of transient duration, and the conspicuous manifestations rarely last more than a few weeks. Particularly, the more florid clinical phenomena are of relatively brief duration, whereas asymmetries in reading and drawing may persist in chronic cases (156). Whereas the hemi-inattentive features clear, the hemianopia and lateralized sensory and motor deficits remain, indicating again that such deficits are not solely responsible for hemi-neglect.

An important feature of hemi-inattention is that the manifestations are selective. Neglect phenomena are variable for stimuli with differing content; neglect is not an all or none phenomenon. A patient may "recognize" his affected limb in one context, but not another. Cohn, Neumann, and Mulder (24) reported the case of a man who, when asked to raise his left arm or leg, invariably raised the right. However, he always pointed correctly to the left side when asked to do so.

Bender, Furlow, and Teuber (14) studied a man with left-sided neglect, who could not recognize familiar people approaching him from the left side, but who responded with a startle reaction to unfamiliar persons coming toward him from that direction. If the hemi-inattentive patient is given a pair of gloves to put on, he most often uses the hitherto neglected hand to put the glove on the good hand, whereas the previously neglected hand remains ungloved.

The selective nature of hemi-neglect is also revealed in the observation that no patient is hemi-inattentive in all respects. Ambulatory patients walk about without colliding into objects or people. Patients omitting the limbs on one side of a figure drawing may center the drawing on the page and may bisect a line correctly. A patient may neglect one half of a visual display, but draw a symmetrical clock. He may respond to some people, but not others, when spoken to from the neglected side. This selectivity is not always the same from day to day. Thus, the manifestations of hemi-inattention cannot be elicited with the same consistency as evidence of sensory or motor deficit alone. This selectivity is illustrated again in the patients' reading. They may ignore one side of an open book, but, in reading a word, they rarely split the midline. When given a word like "clever" they may read "lever" or "ever," but never "ver." They omit only enough to leave a meaningful residue. Thus, one of our subjects read the headline:

10 HOSTAGES HELD IN BROOKLYN
POLICE PREPARED FOR LONG WAIT
as
HOSTAGES HELD IN BROOKLYN FOR LONG WAIT.

This last observation indicates an important feature of hemi-inattention: its manifestations show not only a deficit, but actually a kind of "attention" to the affected side. This was shown dramatically by one man with left-sided neglect who, when asked to draw a daisy, placed petals only on the right side. He then proceeded to rotate the page in a clockwise fashion, all the time continuing to fill in petals on the right side until a full circle of petals was reached. The positive features of hemi-inattention are well illustrated in drawings, which can be highly artistic and symbolic of events on one side of the body and space. In a human figure drawing, the members that are omitted or distorted or caricatured are the mirror images of the patient's own affected side. A patient with a left hemiparesis drew the figure of a man holding his (right) arm behind his body, out of sight. A man with a visual field defect drew a closed window on the corresponding side of a house. A man with left-sided hemi-inattention drew one side of the body with a heavy line, and the affected side of the body was barely visible (Fig. 1). Actions may also be exquisitely selective and symbolic. One woman would expose only her left breast; a man would sit only on one buttock. Another patient, when putting on his eyeglasses, placed the lens correctly in front of his good eye but

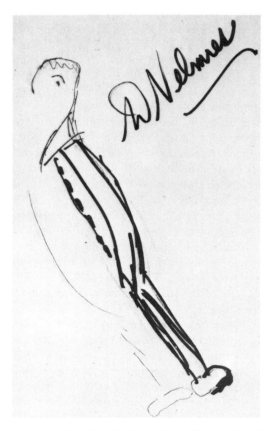

FIG. 1. Human figure drawing of hemi-inattentive patient with considerable artistic talent. Note the "awareness" of the affected side indicated by the lightly penciled line.

over the eyebrow on his affected side. In summary, the syndromes of hemi-neglect have positive as well as negative features.

EXTINCTION AND PATTERNS OF PERCEPTUAL RIVALRY

Extinction on tactile and/or visual double simultaneous stimulation (DSS) occurs in almost all patients with hemi-inattention, but the relationship of extinction to other manifestations of hemi-neglect remains a subject of debate.

The method of DSS was first mentioned in 1884 by Jacques Loeb (16). Oppenheim (94) found tactile extinction on DSS and Anton (3) recorded visual defects on DSS. In 1917, Poppelreuter (104) demonstrated homonymous visual defects elicitable on double, but not on single, stimulation. Poppelreuter referred to this phenomenon as "visual inattention" and "hemianopic weakness of attention." The technique of DSS was reintroduced into neurological examination by Bender (10) and Critchley (26). Bender considered extinction and its sensory analogs under the rubric of perceptual rivalry. In addition to extinction and displacement, he described exosomesthesia, a displacement of one of the two stimuli into extrapersonal space (120). One stimulus may be felt to be of less intensity (obscuration). Both stimuli may be perceived initially, but with continued application, extinction may occur on one side (altered adaptation time). Also, there is a variable period of seconds before the extinguished stimulus is perceived after the removal of the stimulation from the normal side.

Extinction on DSS may be elicited using touch, pin prick, auditory, visual, graphesthesic, stereognostic, gustatory (10), vibratory (26), and barognostic stimuli (54). Cross-modal interactions may be tested with a combination of visual-auditory, visual-tactile, or auditory-tactile stimuli. Cross-modal interactions are seen almost exclusively in those patients with organic mental impairment. In addition, extinction on auditory stimulation appears to be less common than in other modalities, and its presence appears to be dependent on mental defects (12).

An oculomotor analog of extinction was described by Cohn (23) in patients with hemianopia. When the examiner presents a hand or some other object simultaneously in each visual field, the patient, without prior instructions to fixate, is asked to say what he sees. There is a marked conjugate deviation to the unaffected side, i.e., side of the lesion, which is so consistent on repetition that Cohn emphasizes its "magnetic" quality. This eye shift is observed in almost all cases of visual hemi-inattention and persists even after it is called to the patient's notice. It occurs even when the patient is asked to fixate, and it may even be apparent when both stimuli are placed in the patient's good visual field. As is the case in sensory extinction, the phenomenon is generally not found on presentation of a single stimulus. The patient is not aware of the eye movement. Almost always, eye shift is associated with visual extinction, but when stimuli are presented simultaneously in the good field, the patient sometimes, along with the eye shift, reports seeing both stimuli.

Another form of perceptual interaction may be seen when a geometrical figure, such as a circle or square, is tachistoscopically exposed with the image falling on both intact and impaired visual fields. Completion of the half circle or square may occur with the patient reporting a full figure. In addition, it occurs with objectively incomplete figures, ruling out residual vision in the impaired field as a possible explanation (155). This completion effect, originally described by Poppelreuter (104), cannot be owing to a shift in fixation, as it occurs under conditions too brief to allow for a shift. A significant relationship has been documented between the incidence of completion and denial of visual field defect (136). New applications of the completion phenomenon to the study of hemisphere interaction in split-brain patients have been developed by J. Levy *(this volume).*

The study of patients with callosal sections has recently provided renewed interest in the phenomenon of perceptual rivalry. Extinction is commonly found after section of the corpus callosum. The laterality and manifestations vary with the modalities tested, the method of testing, the time elapsed since the operation, and the type of and extent of extracallosal brain damage. Eidelberg and Schwartz (40) have demonstrated that callosal section does not prevent the subsequent production of tactile extinction by posterior parietal lesions in monkeys. In the auditory sphere, left-ear stimuli are extinguished with dichotic presentation of words or digits in normals. Right-ear stimuli are extinguished (left-ear preference) with dichotically presented melodies (73), familiar environmental noises (30), and unintelligible sounds (123). Milner et al. (88) have reported that the "lateralized suppression" of digits presented dichotically is increased in split-brain patients. They found that these patients could report very few of the digits reaching the left ear in the dichotic situation. Other examples of hemisphere specialization and interaction are discussed by M. Kinsbourne, J. Levy, and R. Joynt *(this volume).* Teng and Sperry (128) reported visual extinction in this task was determined by the site of preexisting, extracallosal brain damage. Bender and Diamond (12) and Goodglass (52) studied patients with lateralized brain lesions and intact corpora callosa and found that auditory extinction to a variety of sounds occurred in the ear contralateral to the lesion. Thus, the laterality of extinction following callosal section depends on the specialization of the hemisphere and the side of the lesion.

All writers agree on the importance of perceptual rivalry in the analysis of hemi-inattention, but the question remains as to the relationship of extinction to the other manifestations of hemi-neglect, such as the ignoring of one side of space and the failure to recognize the limbs on the affected side. Critchley (26) states that "the phenomenon of tactile inattention is probably yet another instance of unilateral neglect brought out by a technique of DSS." Denny-Brown (32) feels that extinction is "the prime feature of hemi-inattention;" Heilman and his associates (61,62) regard extinction and hemi-neglect as identical. Battersby, Bender, Pollack, and Kahn (9) believe that the more conspicuous manifestations of unilateral neglect are not those of extinction alone, but occur only in the presence of an organic mental syndrome involving bilateral brain dysfunction. Weinstein and Friedland *(this volume)* claim that, whereas unimodal extinction and eye shift may exist with a normal mental state, cross-modal extinction and the positive conspicuous manifestations of hemi-neglect occur only in association with disturbances of mood and consciousness.

ASSOCIATED DISTURBANCES OF BEHAVIOR

Denial of illness, or anosognosia, in its various forms, is probably the most commonly observed behavioral disturbance seen in association with unilateral neglect. The early writers did not differentiate sharply between anosognosia or verbal denial of illness and the nonverbal aspects of hemi-neglect, and described cases of denial of many types of disability. Lack of recognition of blindness, or Anton's syndrome, was actually first noted by Von Monakow (134). Anton (3) emphasized the relationship of unawareness of disease and focal cerebral lesions. Pick (98) first reported unawareness of hemiplegia. Babinski (5,6) and Babinski and Joltrain (7) coined the term "anosognosia," literally, lack of knowledge of disease, to describe two patients with unawareness of a left hemiplegia. One would ignore commands to move her left hand, and the other stated that she was not paralyzed. When asked what her trouble was she gave "pain in the back" and "phlebitis" as the difficulty. When requested to move her left arm, she either did not respond or said, "Voilà, c'est fait." Babinski noted that the anosognosia may be of short duration as compared to the hemiplegia itself. Marie (84) contributed to an extension of the concept, pointing out the lack of awareness of hemianopia resulting from cerebral lesions.

Since that time, the manifestations of denial have been widely documented. Patients may not only explicitly deny that there is anything wrong with the affected side, but may evade and minimize. This may be illustrated by the patient with a left hemiplegia, who, when asked, "What is your main trouble? Why are you in the hospital?", responds with, "My sister thought I should come in for some tests. I'm hungry. When can I eat?" When asked specifically about the plegic left arm, such a patient may report, "The arm is just a little stiff from arthritis. It will be all better soon." These patients do not learn from experience and may reject all evidence of their disability as inconsequential. Patients with implicit denial may fail to answer when questioned about the affected side or may respond with dysarthric speech after a marked delay and may demonstrate ludic or euphoric behavior. Also, patients with anosognosia, as mentioned, may deny other disabilities and aspects of illness, such as blindness, incontinence, involuntary movements, aphasia, and the fact of an operation. They may deny that they are ill at all. Interestingly, these patients, despite their denial, remain in the hospital and cooperate in examinations, laboratory investigations, and even surgery (144). Such misconceptions include the idea that the limbs do not belong to the patient, and that they are the property of someone else, usually the doctor or a relative. Confabulations in which the affected side is represented in metaphorical or allegorical language may be quite elaborate. Weinstein, Cole, Mitchell, and Lyerly (141) reported the case of a patient with a right hemiparesis, inattention to his right side, and dysphasia, who told the fictitious story that he had been riding in an open truck (in the winter) when his right side became frozen. He said he tried to call to the driver inside the cab to stop, but the driver was unable to understand him because of the noise of the engine.

The affected side of the body and/or space may also be symbolically represented in figures of speech, such as metaphor, simile, personification, metonymy, irony, slang, and humor. A hemiparetic patient repeatedly expressed the conviction that the city should remit one-half of the taxes on his home because of depreciation. Critchley (29) describes patients who referred to their affected extremities in such terms as "silly Jimmy," "sloppy Joe," "Fanny Ann," "the stinker," or "a piece of dead meat." One of his patients called his paralyzed arm "the communist" because it refused to work. Critchley also noted that patients might express anger at the impaired extremity, striking it or screaming abuse at it. He termed this behavior "misoplegia" or morbid hatred of hemiplegia.

Hemi-inattentive patients not infrequently refer to themselves and their affected limbs in the third syntactical person, as did Hughlings Jackson's patient. They are more likely to say *"it* doesn't move the way I want it to" or *"he* doesn't move" than "I have trouble in raising my arm." Similarly, they may say "the *doctor* says there is something wrong." Patients with ludic behavior often use the second syntactical person, referring to the examiner's health or vision when asked how they feel or how well they see. This language suggests that the patient senses the affected part of the body as outside of himself.

Other disorders of behavior commonly associated with conspicuous unilateral neglect are disorientation for place and time, reduplication for place, time, and persons, and nonaphasic misnaming (144). As is the case with the manifestations of hemi-neglect itself, all of these disturbances do not present themselves in all patients. Patients with very marked mood changes, such as highly ludic and euphoric attitudes or withdrawal states, may retain orientation and name objects properly.

In disorientation for place, the patient misnames and mislocates the hospital, or greatly condenses the distance between the hospital and his home (96). In misnaming, the patient usually gives the name of some other hospital, most often located near his home or his place of occupation. At times, the name given to the hospital symbolizes the patient's problems, as in the case of the patient, cited by Weinstein and Friedland *(this volume),* who referred to the "Veterans Armless Hospital." As in the instance of hemi-inattention itself, the patient usually persists in his error even after his attention has been called to it. Weinstein and Kahn (143) have noted that a patient may continue to misname the hospital, even though the name is displayed in plain view. As Hughlings Jackson (66) stated, disorientation for place cannot be attributed to "confusion," unless one were to say that the patient is specifically confused only for the name of the hospital.

In disorientation for date, the patient gives the wrong month and year, and in disorientation for time of day the patient may give an afternoon hour in the morning or vice versa. As in disorientation for place, the presence of a watch does not prevent the patient from remaining disoriented, as the patient does not consult it or use the cues and clues in the environment through which he might orient himself.

Reduplication is closely related to disorientation. In reduplication for place, the patient usually states that there are two or more hospitals of the same or similar names. The phenomenon was originally described by Pick (99), who termed it "reduplicative paramnesia." He described the case of a patient with senile dementia, who, while in Pick's clinic in Prague, said that she had been in another clinic in another city, although the two clinics were exactly alike and a professor of the same name headed each clinic. In reduplication for person, the patient assigns two or more identities to the same person. An example given by Weinstein and Kahn (144) is of a patient who believed that he was being nursed by a mother and daughter, with the "mother" coming one day and the "daughter" on alternate days. Temporal reduplication is closely related to reduplication for persons and is actually an enduring déjà vu experience. Thus, a patient may claim that he has previously been examined by his hospital doctor in the doctor's private office. There may also be reduplication for body parts in which the patient claims that he has two left arms or legs, or even more than one head. Although the fictitious hospital, person, or body part closely resembles the original, it usually differs in some way that is germane to the patient's problems. Thus, the "extra" hospital may be a convalescent place that does not take serious cases, or it may be close to the patient's home. The "extra" arm may be perfectly healthy. It should be pointed out that such patients are not "psychotic" or manifestly "confused," and that they usually make these statements in a matter of fact way. Much of the time the statements are not volunteered, and, to elicit them, the examiner must ask specific questions. This is largely the reason why the phenomena of reduplication are not more generally found and reported.

In nonaphasic misnaming, the patient selectively misnames objects connected with illness and areas of personal identity. Weinstein and Kahn (143) and Geschwind (48) have pointed out that these are not aphasic errors. As with the features of hemi-inattention itself, the misnaming is selective and responds poorly to correction. For example, patients refer to a wheelchair as a "stroller" and bedrails as a "starting gate."

The mood changes are those of indifference and apathy, depression and withdrawal, euphoria and ludic behavior, and paranoid attitudes (144,146,147). Actually, singular indifference and lack of interest have been observed by many writers, but they have not regarded the behavior as an integral part of the hemi-neglect syndrome. The mood changes cover a wide area ranging from the alert, comic attitude of some patients to states of marked withdrawal presenting a picture of akinetic mutism (146). These withdrawn patients move little and speak rarely, or when they do, talk in barely audible sounds. They ignore the affected side by turning the head and eyes to the opposite side, failing to respond to stimuli on one side and failing to respond to questions about the affected side. Not uncommonly, such patients display generalized pain asymbolia. Weinstein and Kahn comment on the mixture of comic and tragic melodramatic behavior that may appear.

Alterations in sexual behavior were noted by Weinstein and Kahn (145) in 9 of 19 patients with marked hemi-inattention. One of their subjects with left-sided neglect conspicuously exposed her left breast. Other changes include verbal and physical sexual advances, open masturbation, attribution of the illness to sexual causes, and delusions and confabulations about sex.

Constructional apraxia may also be found in hemi-inattentive patients. Constructional apraxia was described first by Kleist (80) as "a disturbance which appears in formative activities (arranging, building, drawing) and in which the spatial part of the task is missed, although there is no apraxia for single movement." It was felt to be associated with left parietal lesions. Paterson and Zangwill (96,97) and McFie, Piercy, and Zangwill (82) documented the occurrence of the disability with right-sided lesions and concluded that "the greater part of the constructional disability can be explained in terms of neglect of the left side of visual space (unilateral spatial agnosia) and a disorganization of discriminative spatial judgment (planotopokinesia)." In a later paper, however, Zangwill (41) no longer felt that an absolute relationship existed between the two disorders.

Hacaen (55,56) has provided quantitative data on the association of constructional apraxia with unilateral spatial agnosia (unilateral neglect) in an analysis of 415 cases with post-Rolandic lesions (Table 1).

Hecaen's figures show the frequent combination of unilateral neglect, constructional apraxia, and dressing apraxia with right cerebral lesions and a significant correlation among unilateral neglect (hemiasomatagnosia), sensory loss, visual field defect, constructional apraxia, and disturbances of consciousness. He has

TABLE 1. *Behavioral manifestations of cerebral lesions**

Constructional apraxia	62% of right lesions
	40% of left lesions
	74% of bilateral lesions
Dressing apraxia	22% of right lesions
	4% of left lesions
	20% of bilateral lesions
Of those with no evidence of unilateral spatial agnosia	37% had sensory loss
	54% had visual field defect
	47% had constructional apraxia
	22% had somatognosia
	27% had disturbance of consciousness
Of those with unilateral spatial agnosia (59 cases)	81% had sensory loss
	76% had visual field defect
	95% had constructional apraxia
	58% had somatognosia
	54% had disturbance of consciousness

* Adapted from Hecaen (refs. 55,56).

also reported a 35% association of dressing apraxia with "unilateral somato-gnosic disorders" and a 51% association with unilateral spatial agnosia (55).

Dressing apraxia, occurring in 22% of Hecaen's cases with right-brain lesions and in 4% of those with left-hemisphere lesions, was originally described by Brain (18) as an isolated form of ideational apraxia. He felt that it was closely related to "the disorder of body scheme for one half of the body, for the recognition of the structure of clothes must necessarily be intimately related to the perception of the body." It should be pointed out, however, that the great majority of Hecaen's patients with unilateral neglect were able to dress themselves, and that dressing apraxia may exist in the absence of hemi-neglect. Also, hemi-inattentive subjects with difficulties in dressing may be unable to deal effectively with both sides of the garment and may have trouble in distinguishing the top from the bottom.

Topographical disorientation may also exist in cases of hemi-neglect with right parietal lobe lesions. Topographical disorientation consisting of difficulty in route finding and confusions of directions and locations on maps was originally described by Willbrand in 1892 (150) with later contributions by Pötzl (105), Holmes (63), and Holmes and Horrax (65). It was originally thought to result primarily from left-sided lesions, but later studies have shown a significant association with right parietal lesions (58). Typically, these patients have trouble with both sides of a map and misplace in both east–west and north–south directions. In losing their way in a familiar environment, such as home or the hospital and their own neighborhoods, they make errors with both left and right turns.

ANIMAL STUDIES

Neglect was produced experimentally in animals before it was well recognized by clinical investigators. David Ferrier (42) found altered temperament in three monkeys with bilateral frontal lobe lesions, along with apathy, somnolence, and an absent "power of attentive observation." The first experimental production of unilateral neglect was accomplished by Bianchi (17), who made unilateral prefrontal lesions in monkeys and dogs, using as his chief guide the electrical reactions of the frontal regions via exploration with an "exciter connected with a Dubois Reymond sledge apparatus" (testing the strength of current on his tongue to maintain the proper intensity of stimulation). His cortical excisions, carried out 2 to 3 mm in front of excitable areas for arm, face, or jaw movements, produced an ipsiversive rotation lasting 1 to 2 weeks and a paresis of the contralateral arm, which was not evident in associated movements (climbing or seizing a stick) but was manifest on more delicate movements. The animal was noted to use the paretic extremity only when the other was immobilized. This motor deficit lasted up to 3 weeks and was accompanied by unresponsiveness to contralateral visual stimuli.

Thus, the characteristic feature of neglect in animals becomes apparent: a behavioral deficit that is not consistent for all tasks and not dependent solely on sensory or motor dysfunction. In addition, on most occasions the lesions producing neglect are not limited to classically accepted primary sensory or motor areas, and the resulting deficits appear to resolve sooner than those resulting from primary sensory or motor lesions. These are essential features of hemi-neglect in man.

Kennard (69) studied the response to visual stimuli of monkeys with frontal lobe lesions and found a visual deficit that was not a true hemianopia. The lack of response to contralateral visual stimuli gradually resolved over a few weeks postsurgery, and bilateral lesions did not result in total blindness. Area 8 was felt to be of greatest importance in the production of this syndrome. The visual deficit was accompanied by deviations of head and eyes to the side of the lesion, and a reluctance to use the contralateral hand was noted, without a detectable paresis. The head and eye deviation was not felt to be responsible for the perceptual deficit, as it was outlasted by the visual disregard.

Welch and Stuteville (149) duplicated the production of unilateral neglect with frontal lesions with strictly limited suction of the cortex in the depth of the posterior part of the superior limb of the arcuate sulcus. The monkeys developed ipsiversive circling, increased by arousal, with unresponsiveness to contralateral visual or tactile stimuli. The head and eyes did not attempt compensation by rotation to the side of visual deficit, as had been seen in monkeys with hemianopias from occipital lesions. On occasion, turning to the good side occurred with auditory stimuli on the side contralateral to the lesion. There was neglect of food placed in the side of the mouth contralateral to the lesion, and a failure to lick peanut butter off that side of the face. The involved extremities were used well in walking and climbing, but not in other activities. The involved arm was found to cross the midline on occasion to ward off stimuli from the uninvolved side (together with the normal arm). Recovery began in 5 to 7 days, and was complete in 2 weeks. Welch and Stuteville concluded that the production of this remarkable syndrome by such a limited lesion must represent the upsetting of a "rather simple event . . . This might be a facilitatory mechanism bearing upon the several receiving areas of the involved hemisphere." This hypothesis is similar to that offered by Ferrier and Turner (43), who proposed that a diaschisis resulting from their frontal lesions was responsible, i.e., "a dynamic influence exerted by the magnitude of the lesion on the sensory centers or tracts, which were not organically injured."

Although the involvement of deeper brain structures, such as the centrencephalic or limbic reticular system, was noted clinically by Weinstein, Kahn, and Slote (146), the first production of hemi-neglect by a brain stem lesion was reported by Sprague and his co-workers (125,126,127). Electrolytic lesions of the lateral brain stem (involving the lemnisci) in cat resulted in contralateral visual, olfactory, tactile, proprioceptive, nociceptive, auditory, and gustatory deficits. Visual loss was found to be homonymous for testing with each eye alone, even though there was no lesion in the visual system itself. The syndrome was felt to result from a form of sensory deprivation, "a failure in the capacity to utilize sensory information in making adaptive responses to the environment, in attending to relevant stimuli, and in localizing stimuli in space or on the body surface." It was suggested by Sprague and his colleagues that the lemniscal lesions deafferented the cerebrum, impairing its function.

Adey (1) produced unilateral neglect contralateral to rostral subthalamic lesions in cats. In an approach to food in a modified T-maze on the basis of a visual cue, the animals consistently failed to approach rewards placed in the field of vision opposite the lesion, whereas rewards placed in the ipsilateral field were detected. The defect was temporary, lasting 7 to 10 days. A second similar lesion in the remaining undamaged thalamic zone was followed by a similar defect. Adey noted that even though the cat would watch the experimenter conceal the food reward in the contralateral field, he would completely ignore that side of the environment, even with delay periods as short as 2 sec. Adey attributed neglect to interference with the rhinencephalic–midbrain pathways in the absence of damage to the lemniscal systems.

The importance of upper brain stem structures in visual processes was further demonstrated by Sprague and Meikle (127) and Sprague (125). Unilateral lesions of the superior colliculus (not involving tegmentum or pretectum) of cats were found to produce a contralateral homonymous visual field defect with neglect and extinction on DSS, along with ipsiversive forced circling, a deficit in contralateral eye movements, and a "heightened compulsive response to ipsilateral stimuli." Mislocalization of contralateral acoustic, tactile, and nociceptive stimuli was also observed. It was determined that the motor defect was produced primarily by tectospinal tract lesions, and the visual neglect by lesions of the brachium of the superior colliculus and parts of the tectothalamic system. Recovery occurred over several weeks postsurgery.

Sprague (125) also investigated the effect of unilateral superior colliculus lesions on the hemianopsia resulting from occipital cortex lesion and found that contralateral colliculus section was associated with return of vision to a previously apparently blind field. This same effect was demonstrable with section of the intercollicular commissure. It was concluded that a diminished level of activity in the superior colliculus ipsilateral to a cortical lesion was largely responsible for the visual deficit. As this appeared to be the result of inhibition from the contralateral superior colliculus, it could be ameliorated by collicular commissure section or lesion of the contralateral colliculus. This dramatic recovery, observable immediately after surgery, was accompanied by a visual deficit contralateral to the side of the new lesion, which was less severe than that seen in cats with tectal lesions only. These valuable observations helped to document the interrelationships involved in the production of neglect and established that the hemianopia following occipital lesions in the cat cannot be understood simply as a loss of that cerebral tissue responsible for visual functioning.

Sprague's (125) results were confirmed in the rat by Kirvel et al. (76), who also found multimodal sensory neglect following unilateral superior collicular section with forced ipsiversive circling. Rats with combined ipsilateral superior colliculus and amygdala section were found to have more crossed orientations (turning away from auditory or tactile stimuli on the neglected side) than those without amygdala lesions (75). Amygdala lesions alone did not produce sensory neglect. It was felt that the ipsiversive circling in these animals may have a sensory basis, partly because of the presence of bilateral grooming at a time when circling was still present (20 days postoperatively).

Extinction and synchiria were produced in monkeys by cortical lesions involving areas receiving afferents from the skin, either via thalamocortical or corticocortical relays by Eidelberg and Schwartz (40). Callosal section did not prevent the subsequent appearance of extinction following posterior parietal lesions. Extinction was also produced by lateral lemniscus–lateral hypothalamic tract lesions in the brainstem, but not with midbrain section of the pyramid, or medial lemniscus or dorsal columns of spinal cord. It was concluded that extinction was a result of asymmetrical input and, thereby, altered activity in the two hemispheres was owing to interference with transmission or processing of tactile information. This proposed role of diminished sensory input as the primary determinant of extinction does not concur with the findings in Welch and Stuteville's animals with small frontal lesions (149).

Reeves and Hagamen (107) have also noted extinction to auditory, olfactory, tactile, and visual stimuli with unilateral neglect contralateral to frontal or midbrain reticular formation lesions in cats. These deficits were maintained up to 18 months and were accompanied by significant EEG changes: small-amplitude, high-frequency asynchronous activity contralateral, and large-amplitude, low-frequency synchronous activity ipsilateral to the lesions.

Sensory neglect has been produced by lateral hypothalamic lesions in rats (86). Absent response to visual, olfactory, tactile, or whisker stimuli was observed contralateral to the lesion. Rapid recovery followed, beginning in 1 week with increased orientation to olfactory stimuli and whisker touch, and later with response to visual stimulation. Tactile responsiveness progressed rostrocaudally. Rats with bilateral lateral hypothalamic lesions were adipsic and aphagic for up to 9 days, the recovery from these defects being correlated with recovery of olfactory and whisker touch responsivity. Grooming of unresponsive rats was noted in this paradigm also.

Heilman and his associates have produced unilateral neglect in monkeys from ablation of the inferior parietal lobule (60), from lesions in the mesencephalic reticular formation (138), and lesions in the cingulate gyrus (137). Heilman *(this volume)* discusses the significance of hemi-neglect arising from such widely scattered anatomical sites.

Unilateral neglect has also been produced by chemical agents. Ungerstedt (131,132) inactivated the nigrostriatal system unilaterally by injections of 6-hydroxydopamine hydrobromide. His rats were unresponsive to contralateral stimuli for 3 to 4 days with deviation of the body to the side of the lesion. Olfactory responsiveness appeared after 6 days, vision started to recover after 18 days in some animals, and tactile responsiveness recovered last. Little recovery was seen in the ipsiversive turning. Bilateral removal of this system via the 6-hydroxydopamine (6-OH DA) technique resulted in adipsia, aphagia, and hypoactivity. Ungerstedt believes that the adipsia and aphagia can be explained by the severe sensory neglect and the lack of exploratory behavior.

A most significant study in monkeys, which is highly relevant to the selective features of hemi-neglect in man, is that of Mountcastle (89). Using evoked potentials, he found populations of cells in the parietal association areas of the monkey, Areas 5 and 7, roughly corresponding to the superior and inferior parietal lobule, that fired only when certain motivated actions were carried out on the contralateral side. Area 5 cells fired only if the movement of the contralateral arm satisfied some appetitive drive, such as securing food, grooming, or touching a switch that brought a liquid reward. There were also special cells in Area 7 that were activated when the monkey fixed his gaze on something of interest, such as food when he was hungry.

Obvious difficulties must be considered in the analysis of this body of animal experiments. Experimentally produced lesions cannot be an exact analogue of the clinical situation. That is, neoplasms or vascular diseases do not damage nervous tissue in a way identical to suction or freezing, and spontaneous lesions limited to focal areas of cortex in man are very uncommon. Further, the neural organization of animals is quite different from that of man, particularly in respect to limbic representation in the cortex.

No significant difference has been documented in the neglect caused by right- or left-sided lesions in animals. It appears to occur with the same frequency with lesions of either side. In fact, no hemisphere specialization of any kind has been well documented in any animal species. Thus, those aspects of hemi-inattention of greatest current interest in relation to hemisphere dominance and interaction cannot be studied well in animal models. Also, a precise definition of the syndrome itself is more difficult to accomplish in animal work.

However, unilateral neglect has been created in animals with lesions from the upper brainstem to the cortex. This work is of great value in the analysis of the neuroanatomical, neurochemical, and neurophysiological factors involved in the neglect syndromes. This animal work has contributed to the evolution of a number of valuable theories regarding the genesis of hemi-inattention in man.

THEORETICAL CONSIDERATIONS

Early theories of extinction and perceptual rivalry were reflected in the nomenclature used for the various manifestations. These included Poppelreuter's (104) "hemianopic weakness of attention," pseudohemianopia (121), tactile ineffectiveness (51), relative hemianopia (129), sensory suppression (109), and sensory eclipse (133). Bender *(this volume)* cites the observation of Hippocrates that "of simultaneous pains in two places, the lesser is obliterated by the greater." Heymans' law of inhibition (1927) that simultaneous stimuli mask each other was quoted frequently in the early literature (27). Goldstein thought that extinction represented a diminished capacity of available nerve energy to respond to two separate stimuli at the same time (27). Lhermitte and de Ajuriaguerra (81) spoke of a general rule of symmetrical stimulation whereby strong stimuli on the good side suppress the attenuated stimuli on the impaired side.

Critchley (26), in his encyclopedic review of the subject, regarded the term "inattention" as the least objectionable. He felt that the term "extinction" suggested incorrectly an active process affecting cerebral perceptual functions. He stated that "tactile inattention in parietal patients is probably no more than an instance of local neglect or disregard, which may be demonstrable at times in many other spheres of consciousness" (27). Critchley felt that the responsible lesion was present in the great majority of cases in the parietal lobe, and concluded that the variability of tactile extinction forced him to accept a "psychological" interpretation for these phenomena. He stated, "The brain injured individual cannot 'attend' to two simultaneous claimant stimuli, to the detriment of the one which is of lesser intensity, or which proceeds from a segment of higher limen, or from regions which have become less obtrusive within the body-scheme." In Critchley's view, the parietal cortex served as an organ of local attention and as a "storehouse of past impressions, and hence, in the handing up of a body scheme or *image de soi;*" the sensory defect produced the perceptual rivalry because of the unequal strength of the double percepts. The result was the phenomenon of inattention.

Bender's work in the 1940s and 1950s was the major impetus to a development of interest in perceptual rivalry (10,13,14). Bender preferred a phenomenological approach to perceptual rivalry, referring to extinction as a "process in which a sensation disappears or becomes imperceptible when another sensation is evoked by simultaneous stimuli elsewhere in the sensory field" (10). He emphasized the value of extinction as a sensitive indication of sensory deficit. In one series of 50 consecutive cases of hemiparesis, 44 were found to have extinction, obscuration, or displacement on the affected side on DSS testing, whereas only 29 had sensory defects to testing with routine single stimuli (11).

Bender emphasized the role of a heightened threshold in the area from which extinction can be obtained and noted that "displacement occurs across a gradient in sensation from an area of high to one of lower threshold of excitability" (10). He extended the concept of perceptual rivalry in emphasizing that all stimuli have an external or "distal" and internal or "proximal" background. This was demonstrated in a study by Bender and Krieger (15), in which intact perception and localization of visual stimuli were achieved in perimetrically blind fields when tested in darkness.

Bender preferred the phenomenological term "extinction" to "inattention." He pointed out that extinction could not be influenced by active "attention" to the stimulated part (10). This observation was not accepted by Critchley (26), but Denny-Brown, who also preferred the term "extinction," felt that no reinforcement of attention could overcome the defect. He believed that extinction represented a loss or diminution of the "biological significance" of the stimulus (34).

Denny-Brown, Meyer, and Horenstein (35) regarded extinction as a manifestation of amorphosynthesis resulting from parietal dysfunction; a "disturbance of synthesis of multiple sensory data," and agreed that it occurred across altered gradients of sensory threshold.

The implications of the study of perceptual rivalry are increasingly relevant to our subject. While the controversies detailed above have continued unabated with persistent vigor, new theories of hemisphere interaction based on a broader interpretation of these phenomena have been developed. A general principle has been proposed: activation of the good hemisphere further impairs the performance of the injured hemisphere. This applies also to other cerebral functions, more complex than the recognition of two percepts appearing simultaneously on either side. These include reading, speech, and calculation. This principle may also be applied to commissurotomized patients (and perhaps also normals) in whom activation of one hemisphere may cause a reduction in the activity of the other. For example, the increased activity of the left hemisphere, associated with right hand movement or especially speech, may cause a perceptual alteration with favoring of the right visual field and reduction in left visual field perception (130). In this regard, Trevarthen (130) has observed the "perceptual erasure" (the patient reports "it's disappeared!") of a goal in the right visual field when left hand response is required in a commissurotomized patient. Further work in this area is reviewed by Levy *(this volume)* and Kinsbourne *(this volume).*

Hughlings Jackson attributed "imperception" to a "defect of speech" as compared to aphasia, which was a "loss of speech." Comparing the left and right posterior lobes, he regarded the right as the leading side for visual ideation, whereas the left was the more automatic side. With words, the situation was reversed with the right the more automatic half, and the left the leading side "for that use of words which is speech." Jackson actually disliked the term "aphasia," as it implied that language functions were confined to the left hemisphere. He considered his patients' inability to name objects, persons, and places as a defect in visual ideation, a function that in some way involved language.

The early writers, such as Babinski (6,7), Dejerine (31), Barré, Morin, and Kaiser (8), and Pinéas (102), stressed the importance of a loss of deep or cortical sensibility, and we have already reviewed the reasons for the inadequacy of this explanation. The idea of a specific localization for anosognosia, and what later was to become known as hemi-neglect, was first put forth by Pick (100). He attributed the behavior to a lesion in the right parietal lobe or right thalamus. Pick conceived of the representation of a three-dimensional image of the body, which, when damaged, caused the contralateral side to drop out of the patient's awareness. Hauptmann (1927) concurred in such a right-sided localization for the body image, and Pinéas (103) and Scheller and Seidemann (114) reported patients with marked inability to perceive objects, persons, and pictures on the left side of the body in the absence of a hemianopia. This body scheme concept was of importance because it offered an explanation of the predominance of right cerebral lesions and emphasized that visual neglect could not be attributed to a hemianopia.

The body scheme concept was expanded by Brain (18), who described three cases of defective visual localization limited to the homonymous half-fields, a phenomenon that he called "visual disorientation." Two of the three complained of the feeling that the side of the body ipsilateral to the hemianopia did not belong to them. Brain was acquainted with the previous description by Holmes (63,64) of patients with bilateral posterior parietal gunshot wounds, who had disturbances in spatial orientation, object localization, topographical memory, and reading. There were also contributions from the German casualties of World War I, as Kleist (78) found errors in grasping and pointing to visual stimuli in the absence of demonstrable visual field defects, which Kleist called "optical ataxia." He also described agnosia for visual space or "space blindness," which he believed resulted from loss of visual memories. Another report was that of Riddoch (108), who found two patients with visual disorientation limited to the right homonymous field "without any limitation of the visual fields for ordinary stimuli or serious disturbance in vision."

Brain's 1941 paper (18) elaborated on these observations. He presented three cases with large right parietooccipital lesions, left homonymous hemianopia, defective left postural sensibility, and errors in right and left discrimination in route finding without a loss of topographical memory. These patients got lost at home by making right instead of left turns but were able to name correctly their own and the examiner's left and right hands. One patient "complained that he did not know where the left side of his body was. He might awaken lying on his left arm and not know where it was, and when eating would hold the fork up in the air without knowing it. He said that the left side of his body felt different from the right side, and as if it were on the right side." These patients did not demonstrate explicit denial. Brain suggested that they suffered from a defect of "spatial orientation . . . inattention to or neglect of the left half of external space . . . with amnesia for the left half of the body."

The significance of these findings was recognized by Brain, who pointed out that most patients with hemianopia may collide into objects but do not get lost in their own homes. In addition, he concluded that the deficit was not related to the visual agnosia of Kleist (78), as the patients were capable of recognizing their errors. He pointed out that "the patient's behavior towards the left half of external space is similar to the attitude adopted towards the left half of the body by some patients in whom awareness of the body is disordered. Since each half of the body is a part of the corresponding half of external space, it is not surprising to find that perception of the body and perception of external space are closely related and subject to similar disorders."

Brain emphasized the importance of the parietal lobe in body awareness, and the relationship of visual localization to body scheme and the "scheme of the external world." The situation in which the patient behaved as if the limbs were not there was referred to as "amnesia for the left half of the body." An analogy was developed between the phenomenon of allesthesia and the choice of right turns by his patient with left hemispatial neglect.

It was Brain's opinion that the body scheme was localized in the parietal lobes, but that it was organized differently in each hemisphere. Thus, a lesion of the left (dominant) parietal lobe resulted in finger agnosia, agraphia, acalculia, and right–left disorientation (Gerstmann's syndrome), whereas damage to the right (nondominant) parietal lobe caused an amnesia and unawareness of the contralateral half of the body and space.

Gerstmann (47) thought that hemi-neglect and anosognosia were manifestations of an amnestic-agnostic disorder of the postural model of the body and that this disturbance of body image was a unitary modality produced by right parietal, optic thalamus, and thalamoparietal lesions. He felt that the closer the lesion was to the cortex, the more there was the likelihood of complex psychological manifestations. Gerstmann also noted that the "receptive, paraphasic, and syntactic" types of aphasia resulting from left parietal lesions may represent yet another instance of unawareness of illness. This observation was to be developed further by Kinsbourne and Warrington (71) and Weinstein, Lyerly, Cole, and Ozer (142) in their studies of jargon aphasia.

Zangwill and his associates (82,96,97) used the term "visual spatial agnosia" to refer to unilateral neglect. Their patients, all with right parietal lesions, showed defective perception of spatial relationships in performance of constructional tasks, and some had topographical disorientation. The authors suggested a specialization in the right occipitoparietal area for visual spatial cognition. They made the important observation that the patterns of visual spatial and constructional disability found in left- and right-sided cases differed, anticipating later work that has verified this finding.

However, in a later paper, Ettlinger, Warrington, and Zangwill (41), it was found that there was no absolute relationship between "unilateral visuospatial agnosia" and constructional disorders. Some cases with constructional defects had no unilateral neglect, whereas others with unilateral neglect made errors on both sides of the design. Tachistoscopic studies revealed that errors of spatial orientation were made even when the presentation was limited to the good hemi-field. These findings disproved the contention that visual constructive disorder is wholly referable to unilateral neglect, but it was thought to be desirable to retain the term "visual spatial agnosia."

Costa, Vaughan, Horowitz, and Ritter (25), investigating the behavioral deficits associated with unilateral visual spatial neglect, used the Raven's Coloured Progressive Matrices. They found that unilateral neglect, or position preference on the test, was greater in cases with right-hemisphere lesions. They also showed that patients with left-hemisphere lesions and neglect showed equally profound visual spatial defects. This study provided additional evidence against the thesis that visuospatial disorders are at the basis of hemi-inattention.

Another approach to the problem was developed by Denny-Brown and associates (32–35). The parietal lobe was thought to "summate" or "synthesize" the spatial dimensions of contralateral stimuli, and *all* defects associated with parietal lesions were felt to be interrelated and ascribed to a unilateral defect in spatial summation, called "amorphosynthesis." Denny-Brown considered extinction, astereognosis, hemispatial difficulty, constructional apraxia, hemi-neglect, topographical disorientation, unilateral dressing difficulty, and anosognosia as manifestations of a "unilateral distortion of perception resulting in a unilateral disorder of behavior at a physiological level" resulting from a cortical lesion of one parietal lobe. Amorphosynthesis was felt to lack the "conceptual character" necessary for a true agnosia and was not regarded by Denny-Brown as a form of body image defect or as a special spatial sense disturbance. It was, in his opinion, a pure disorder of spatial summation resulting from faulty perception of the spatial aspects of all sensory modalities on one side. The special vulnerability of percepts from the affected side to rivalry with other stimuli was of great importance in the genesis of the symptomatology. Anosognosia, as a manifestation of amorphosynthesis, was seen as the result of the defective synthesis of multiple sensory information from one side, and as a "mental aversion rather than a repression, a mental 'avoiding response' " comparable to the motor avoiding responses seen in these patients. As this was a pure sensory disorder, Denny-Brown noted its occurrence on both sides and felt that no special role could be assumed for the right hemisphere in visual space perception. Aphasia was thought to limit the occurrence of amorphosynthesis with left-sided lesions.

A motivational theory of anosognosia was proposed by Schilder (116), who had reported a case of denial of right hemiplegia in 1932. He pointed out the primary instinctive urge toward maintenance of body integrity governing the patient's behavior and considered denial to be a form of "organic repression." Similar views were developed by Goldstein (51), who felt that denial represented a psychological defence mechanism present in normal individuals, and not necessarily created by brain damage. In Goldstein's view, a "drive to self-actualization" was involved in the production of denial. Sandifer (113) also pointed out the value of denial to the patient in the avoidance of a catastrophic reaction to the stress of disability. Support for this approach was gained from the work of Weinstein and Kahn (144), who noted that patients who developed explicit denial under the necessary conditions of altered brain function were compulsive, perfectionistic people who had, in their premorbid behavior, denied problems and incapacities. These motivational theories, however, had an outstanding fault, in that they did not explain the predominance of right-hemisphere over left-hemisphere lesions in both unilateral neglect and verbal anosognosia.

Denny-Brown and many of the body image and visuospatial agnosia theorists do not attach particular significance to the disorders of mood and consciousness associated with hemi-neglect. Critchley (27), although regarding unilateral neglect and lack of spontaneous movements of the limbs on one side as a manifestation of a parietal lobe lesion, noted the transient nature of denial and its association with a clouded sensorium. A number of authors were impressed by the amnesia, disorientation, and confabulation. In 1908, Redlich and Bonvicini (106) called denial of blindness a Korsakoff syndrome occurring in a blind person. Sandifer (113) stated that anosognosia for hemiplegia could occur with a lesion at any level of the central nervous system, provided that there was an accompanying defect in intellectual function.

Battersby, Bender, Pollack, and Kahn (9), in an often quoted study, believed that hemi-inattention or, as they preferred to call it, unilateral spatial deficit, was caused by a sensory deficit with a background of an organic mental syndrome. They agreed with Denny-Brown that because of the multiple sensory defects and the associated mental deficits, the spatial disorders could not be classified as agnosias or "associational" defects. The authors investigated 85 patients with unilateral localizable space-occupying lesions of either cerebral hemisphere. The criterion for hemi-neglect or "unilateral spatial defect" was a clear, consistent asymmetry on two or more of a series of nine visual, constructional, drawing, geographical, reading, and behavioral tests; in effect, hemi-inattention over and above tactile or visual extinction. Of the subjects with hemi-neglect, as determined by these indices, 80% had nondominant hemisphere lesions and 20% had lesions of the dominant hemisphere. When untestable aphasic patients were included, the proportion was 48% to 40%. The authors interpreted this finding as showing that the proportionate incidence of unilateral spatial deficit did not differ significantly with side of lesion. They found that temporooccipital, parietooccipital, and frontoparietal lesions could all produce the syndrome. All of the patients with unilateral neglect had a hemianopia, and 83% had a somatosensory defect. Although 98% of the subjects with unilateral neglect had disorientation for place and/or time, none of the hemianopic patients in the group without neglect were disoriented.

The Battersby, Bender, Kahn, and Pollack paper (9) confirmed previous observations that hemi-inattention could appear with significant frequency with lesions of the dominant hemisphere and that it was not an occasional finding, like aphasia with a right-hemisphere lesion. Their theory, as is pointed out by Bender *(this volume),* is that sensory extinction is a manifestation of perceptual rivalry and that the unbalance becomes more marked as a result of the superimposed mental deficit. During the completion of visuospatial and constructive tasks, the process appears as hemi-neglect or unilateral spatial deficit.

There is ample evidence that there is a bilateral disturbance in brain function in cases of hemi-neglect. De Renzi and his associates (36,37) found impairment of tactile performance in the good hands of patients with unilateral neglect. They suggested that neglect of space was not directly linked to sensory loss or poor visual scanning, but to a "cognitive defect, which may be viewed as a mutilated representation of space." The study supported the view that hemi-inattention is not wholly explicable on a deficit limited to a single hemisphere.

Clinical pathological studies have shown that in man, as well as in monkeys and cats, the lesions are not confined to the parietal lobes. Weinstein and Kahn believed that a lesion anywhere in the limbic reticular system could be associated with unilateral neglect. Heilman et al. (62,137) subsequently reported cases with cingulate gyrus and frontal lobe lesions. Precise anatomical localization is difficult, even with modern radiographic techniques. Even at autopsy, the site and extent of the lesion may not correlate exactly with the behavior, as the patient may have shown conspicuous signs of neglect only during the early stages of the illness. Unilateral neglect occurs much more often with infiltrating, rapidly developing tumors than with benign masses. It appears particularly after acute vascular lesions, especially when there is subarachnoid bleeding. Neglect does not occur after cortical ablations, indicating that involvement of deeper structures is a necessary condition. Interestingly, according to Smith (122), extinction can be demonstrated after hemispherectomy, but the more conspicuous signs of unilateral neglect do not occur. There is also electrographic evidence that a diffuse disturbance of brain function is involved, in that cases of frank neglect have slow wave activity over the entire affected hemisphere, often with bilateral activity (144).

Weinstein and associates (139–148) have emphasized the positive, adaptive, conceptual, and symbolic aspects of anosognosia and unilateral neglect, as has Critchley (29). They differentiate sensory extinction from the more severe and conspicuous and less enduring aspects of hemi-inattention. They consider that the manifestations of unilateral neglect are, in part, the *gestures* in which the patient symbolizes the affected side, similar to the way he conceptualizes it verbally in delusions, confabulations, humor, and various other forms of metaphorical speech. Weinstein believes that not only are the manifestations of conspicuous neglect invariably associated with disorders of mood and/or consciousness, but that the more colorful signs of unilateral neglect themselves are aspects of a disturbance of consciousness. Although the patient does not consciously express awareness of one side of the body and space, he "unconsciously" displays knowledge in his gestures, emotional attitudes, and such expressions as "dummy," "dopey," "my poor little daughter," and the various examples of misoplegia cited by Critchley (29).

Weinstein and Kahn believe that premorbid personality factors are important, not in the appearance of hemi-inattention per se but in the content of the verbal and nonverbal manifestations. For example, they noted that the personality background of patients who developed hemi-inattention and showed marked withdrawal and pain asymbolia, symbols of death and violence, such as silence and immobility had been prominent, and outbursts of physical violence and temper had been habitual modes of adaptation to stress. The authors labeled these types of hemi-neglect as unilateral akinetic mutism and akinetic mutism as bilateral hemi-inattention (146). Other patients with hemi-neglect were emotionally labile and highly ludic. They referred to the affected limbs in humorous fashion and introduced comic elements into their drawings. The premorbid background of these subjects was described as "emotional," "easily hurt," "warm," "imaginative," and "sympathetic." It was of interest that patients in this group, in their figure drawings, portrayed the other sex and conceptualized the events of their environment in sexual terms.

Kinsbourne (74) has proposed a thesis based on the idea that activation of one hemisphere causes an inhibition of potentially homologous functions in the other hemisphere. When the dominant left hemisphere is verbally activated, in the course of examination of the patient, there is a rightward orientation, including a shift of the eyes to the right, and reduced attention to the left side of space. This is an attractive theory because it explains the predominance of left-sided neglect, and imparts a unitary formation of the various sensory, motor, and directional components of hemi-neglect.

A great deal of recent research on hemi-inattention has been done by K. Heilman and associates *(this volume)* who regard hemi-neglect as a defect in the orienting response or alerting-arousal reaction caused by a lesion anywhere in the corticolimbic reticular loop. This would explain the appearance of neglect in many areas not contiguous to one another. Heilman believes that patients with unilateral neglect have their major dysfunction in the inferior parietal lobule (61), a secondary sensory association area, accounting for the multimodal character of conspicuous neglect. Heilman's work has, as yet, not explained the predominance in man of right-hemisphere lesions.

A major consideration in the evaluation of a theory of hemi-inattention is its explanation of the predominance of neglect of the left side of the body and speech, and it is important to emphasize that no animal experiments have shown such a laterality. The hypothesis that the body image is organized differently in each parietal lobe has been presented, and it has a number of shortcomings. Geschwind (49) has pointed out that lesions of the right parietal lobe affect only the image of the left side of the body, and one would ask where and how the scheme for the right side of the body is organized. Second, the body scheme hypothesis does not explain why patients may not only remain unaware of the limbs on one side of the body, but of other aspects of illness, such as a craniotomy involving the head on the side of the lesion. Third, it does not take into account the fact that patients may be unaware of the affected limbs in one context and not in another; and, finally, it ignores the role of hemisphere interaction.

Paul Schilder (116) suggested that the predominance of right-hemisphere lesions might be due to the exaggeration of a normal trend to left hand subordination. Roth (110) thought that the left side of the body had a "special vulnerability" because of the predominant use of the right hand in dextrals. Hecaen and associates (55–58) have drawn on the work of Semmes, Weinstein, Ghent, and Teuber (119), who, on the basis of a study of the effects of missile wounds, concluded that there was a more diffuse concentration of tactile, perceptual function in the right hemisphere. Hecaen states that the left hemisphere possesses a "more highly differentiated and more homogeneous functional organization," whereas the right hemisphere "appears to be both looser and more labile with regard to appreciation of the body in space."

Another explanation, originally put forth by Nielsen (91) and advanced by Battersby, Bender, Kahn, and Pollack (9), is that the predominance of right-hemisphere lesions is more apparent than real because so many of the subjects with left-hemisphere lesions are aphasic and cannot comprehend tests involving visual search and constructive skills. It is true that, as Gerstmann observed, when people with unilateral neglect are clinically aphasic, they frequently have jargon. Such patients are often very difficult to test, not only because of their defects in comprehension, which vary greatly, but because of their marked disturbances in behavior, which impair their cooperation in many tests. However, the presence of aphasia per se does not interfere with such manifestations of hemi-neglect as eye shift, failure to notice people on one side of a room or food on one side of a plate, inability to imitate the examiner's grasping of both his ears, and omitting a sleeve or slipper on one side in dressing. Moreover, findings after hemispherectomy (122) and callosal section indicate that the right, nondominant hemisphere has a significant degree of auditory comprehension as well as a respectable vocabulary (151).

Weinstein and Cole (140) have explained the predominance of right- over left-hemisphere lesions on the basis of the relative inability of the damaged left hemisphere to use metaphorical speech and gesture and the specialized role of the right hemisphere in integrating the semantic aspects of language with perceptual and emotional processes. These views will be presented more fully by E. A. Weinstein and R. P. Friedland *(this volume)*.

It has been suggested that there is a right hemisphere predominance for emotion in the sense that the left hemisphere is dominant for language. In cases with cerebral lesions, this is based on the evidence that conspicuous hemi-neglect in which mood changes are prominent occurs predominantly with right-hemisphere pathology. In normal subjects, a left-ear superiority has been noted for nonspeech sounds, such as crying, laughing, or coughing (70), and for nonverbal emotionally charged human voices, using nonverbal methods of reporting (19). Using the paradigm developed by Kinsbourne (72), Schwartz et al. (118) found that normal subjects tend to look to the left when answering affectively tinged questions, a tendency increased by spatial factors and diminished by verbal manipulation. These results await more complete verification, but they indicate an exciting area of research highly germane to the phenomena of hemi-neglect.

Experiments on the effects of section of the corpus callosum in man have given a great impetus to problems of hemisphere specialization and interaction, and will be discussed by J. Levy and R. Joynt *(this volume)*. The most spectacular demonstration of hemi-neglect following corpus callosum section appears in a film shown by Gazzaniga (46). A woman to whom a sexy pin-up was flashed in the left field of vision, stated that she saw nothing, but giggled in an unmistakable fashion. Similarly, Zaidel (154) exposed the picture of a tired housewife leaning on a broom to the left visual field of a callosally sectioned patient. When asked to name it she said only that "this is funny, look at this dumbbell." "Dumbbell" was a favorite expression of her husband's. When pressed to describe the picture she said "this is ＿＿" (her husband's nickname). This is an example of the recognition of a metaphorical, self-referential equivalent by the right hemisphere and the transfer of an "emotional" message from the right hemisphere.

The subject of hemi-inattention is, thus, not only of phenomenological and clinical interest, but its history reflects the development of conceptions of neurological function and relationships among perceptual, conceptual, emotional, and linguistic processes. It is well suited as a vehicle for our increasing knowledge in the area of hemisphere specialization and interaction.

ACKNOWLEDGMENT

Research conducted by Robert Friedland was supported in part by Public Health Service Grant #5TOINS-05072.

REFERENCES

1. Adey, W. R., Walter, D. O., and Lindsley, D. F. (1962): Subthalamic lesions. *Arch. Neurol.,* 6:194–207.
2. Albert, M. L. (1973): A simple test of visual neglect. *Neurology (Minneap.),* 23:658–664.
3. Anton, G. (1899): Ueber die selbstwahmehmungen der herderkankungen des Gehirns durch den Kranken bei Rindenblindheit und Rindentaubheit. *Arch. Psychiatr. Nervenkr.,* 32:86–127.
4. Babenkova, S. V. (1976): The syndrome of "pseudomoria" and its relation to disorder of body scheme in right hemisphere stroke patients. In: *Cerebral Vascular Disease, Seventh International Conference, Salzburg,* edited by J. S. Meyer, H. Lechner, and M. Reivich. Thieme Publ., Stuttgart.
5. Babinski, J. (1914): Contribution à l'étude des troubles mentaux dans l'hémiplégie organique cérébrale (anosognosie). *Rev. Neurol. (Paris),* 27:845–848.
6. Babinski, J. (1918): Anosognosie. *Rev. Neurol. (Paris),* 25:365–367.
7. Babinski, J., and Joltrain, E. (1924): Un nouveau cas d'anosognosie. *Rev. Neurol. (Paris),* 31:638–640.
8. Barré, J. A., Morin, L., and Kaiser (1923): Etude clinique d'un nouveau cas d'anosognosie de Babinski. *Rev. Neurol. (Paris),* 39:500–504.
9. Battersby, W. S., Bender, M. B., Pollack, M., and Kahn, R. L. (1956): Unilateral "spatial agnosia" (inattention) in patients with cerebral lesions. *Brain,* 79:68–93.
10. Bender, M. B. (1952): *Disorders in Perception.* Charles C Thomas, Springfield, Ill.
11. Bender, M. B. (1970): Perceptual interactions. In: *Modern Trends in Neurology,* edited By Denis Williams, pp. 1–28. Butterworths, London.
12. Bender, M. B., and Diamond, S. P. (1965): An analysis of auditory perceptual defects. *Brain,* 88:675–686.
13. Bender, M. B., and Furlow, L. T. (1945): Phenomenon of visual extinction in homonymous fields and psychologic principles involved. *Arch. Neurol. Psychiatry,* 53:29–33.
14. Bender, M. B., Furlow, L. T., and Teuber, H. L. (1949): Alterations in behavior after massive cerebral trauma (intraventricular foreign body). *Confin. Neurol.,* 9:140–157.
15. Bender, M. B., and Krieger, H. P. (1951): Visual functions in perimetrically blind fields. *Arch. Neurol. Psychiatry,* 65:72–79.
16. Benton, A. L. (1956): Jacques Loeb and the method of double stimulation. *J. Hist. Med.,* 11:47–53.
17. Bianchi, L. (1895): The functions of the frontal lobes. *Brain,* 18:497–522.
18. Brain, W. R. (1941): Visual disorientation with special reference to lesions of the right cerebral hemisphere. *Brain,* 64:244–272.
19. Carmon, A., and Nachson, I. (1973): Ear asymmetry in perception of emotional non-verbal stimuli. *Acta Psychol.,* 37:351–357.

20. Cibis, P., and Muller, H. (1948): Lokaladaptometrische Untersuchungen am Projektionsperimeter nach Maggiore. *Arch. Ophthamol.,* 148:468–489.
21. Cobb, S. (1947): Amnesia for the left limbs developing into anosognosia. *Bull. Los Angeles Neurol. Soc.,* 12:48–52.
22. Cohn, R. (1961): *The Person Symbol in Clinical Medicine.* Charles C Thomas, Springfield, Ill.
23. Cohn, R. (1972): Eyeball movements in homonymous hemianopia following simultaneous bitemporal object presentation. *Neurology (Minneap.),* 22:12–14.
24. Cohn, R., Neumann, M., and Mulder, D. W. (1948): Anosognosia. *Q. Rev. Psychiatry Neurol.,* 3:83.
25. Costa, L. D., Vaughan, H. G., Jr., Horowitz, M., and Ritter, W. (1969): Patterns of behavioral deficit associated with unilateral spatial neglect. *Cortex,* 59:242–263.
26. Critchley, M. (1949): The phenomenon of tactile inattention with special reference to parietal lesions. *Brain,* 72:538–561.
27. Critchley, M. (1953): *The Parietal Lobes.* Hafner, New York.
28. Critchley, M. (1955): Personification of paralyzed limbs in hemiplegics. *Br. Med. J.,* 30:284.
29. Critchley, M. (1974): Misoplegia or hatred of hemiplegia. *Mt. Sinai J. Med.,* 41:82–87.
30. Curry, F. K. W. (1967): A comparison of left handed and right handed subjects on verbal and non-verbal listening tasks. *Cortex,* 3:343–352.
31. Dejerine, J. (1914): in discussion of paper by Babinski, J. (1914): Contribution à l'études des troubles mentaux dans l'hemiplegie organique cérébrale (anosognosie). *Rev. Neurol. (Paris),* 27:845–848.
32. Denny-Brown, D. (1963): The physiological basis of perception and speech. In: *Problems of Dynamic Neurology,* edited by L. Halpern. Jerusalem Post Press, Jerusalem.
33. Denny-Brown, D., and Banker, B. Q. (1954): Amorphosynthesis from left parietal lesions. *Arch. Neurol.,* 71:302–313.
34. Denny-Brown, D., and Chambers, R. A. (1958): The parietal lobe and behavior. *Res. Publ. Assoc. Res. Nerv. Ment. Dis.,* 36:35–117.
35. Denny-Brown, D., Meyer, J. S., and Horenstein, S. (1952): The significance of perceptual rivalry. *Brain,* 75:433–471.
36. DeRenzi, E., and Faglioni, P. (1967): The relationship between visuospatial impairment and constructional apraxia. *Cortex,* 3:327–342.
37. DeRenzi, E., Faglioni, P., and Scotti, G. (1970): Hemispheric contribution to exploration of space through the visual and tactile modality. *Cortex,* 6:191–203.
38. Duke-Elder, W. S. (1949): *Textbook of Ophthalmology. Vol. 4: The Neurology of Vision, Motor and Optical Anomalies.* Mosby, London.
39. Ehrenwald, H. (1931): Anosognosie und Depersonalisation. *Nervenarzt,* 4:681–688.
40. Eidelberg, E., and Schwartz, A. S. (1971): Experimental analysis of the extinction phenomenon in monkeys. *Brain,* 94:91–108.
41. Ettlinger, G., Warrington, E., and Zangwill, O. L. (1957): A further study of visual-spatial agnosia. *Brain,* 80:335–361.
42. Ferrier, D. (1876): *The Functions of the Brain.* Putnam's Sons, New York.
43. Ferrier, D., and Turner, W. A. (1898): *Phil. Trans. R. Soc. Lond. [Biol.],* 190:1–3.
44. Fisher, C. M. (1956): Hemiplegia and motor impersistence. *J. Nerv. Ment. Dis.,* 122:20.
45. Furmanski, A. R. (1950): The phenomena of sensory suppression. *Arch. Neurol. Psychiatry,* 63:205–217.
46. Gazzaniga, M. S. (1970): *The Bisected Brain.* Appleton-Century Crofts, New York.
47. Gerstmann, J. (1942): Problem of imperception of disease and of impaired body territories with organic lesions. *Arch. Neurol. Psychiatry,* 48:890–913.
48. Geschwind, N. (1964): Non-aphasic disorders of speech. *Int. J. Neurol.,* 4:207–214.
49. Geschwind, N. (1970): in discussion of Kinsbourne, M. (1970): A model for the mechanism of unilateral neglect of space. *Trans. Am. Neurol. Assoc.,* 95:143–146.
50. Geschwind, N. (1974): The anatomical basis of hemispheric differentiation. In: *Hemisphere Function in the Human Brain,* edited by S. J. Dimond and J. G. Beaumont. ELEK Science, London.
51. Goldstein, K. (1939): *The Organism, a Holistic Approach to Biology Derived from Pathological Data in Man.* American Book Co., New York.
52. Goodglass, H. (1967): Binaural digit presentation and early lateral brain damage. *Cortex,* 3:295–306.

53. Grunbaum, A. A. (1930): Ueber Apraxie (mit Filmvorführrrungen). *Zbl. Ges. Neurol. Psychiatr.,* 55:788–792. [Quoted by Critchley, M. (1953): *The Parietal Lobes.* Hafner Press, New York.]
54. Head, H., and Holmes, G. (1911): Sensory disturbances from cerebral lesions. *Brain,* 34:102–254.
55. Hecaen, H. (1962): Clinical symptomatology of right and left hemisphere lesions. In: *Interhemispheric Relations and Cerebral Dominance,* edited by V. B. Mountcastle. Johns Hopkins Press, Baltimore, Md.
56. Hecaen, H. (1969): Aphasic, apraxic and agnosic syndromes in right and left hemisphere lesions. In: *Disorders of Speech, Perception and Symbolic Behavior, Handbook of Neurology, Volume 4,* edited by P. J. Vinken and G. W. Bruyn. North Holland, Amsterdam.
57. Hecaen, H., and Angelerques, R. (1963): *La Cécité Psychique.* Masson, Paris. [Quoted by Gainotti, G. (1972): Emotional behavior and hemispheric side of the lesion. *Cortex,* 8:41–55.]
58. Hecaen, H., Penfield, W., Bertrand, C., and Malmo, R. (1956): The syndrome of apractognosia due to lesions of the minor hemisphere. *Arch. Neurol. Psychiatry,* 75:400–434.
59. Heilman, K. M., Pandya, D. N., and Geschwind, N. (1970): Trimodal inattention following parietal lobe ablations. *Trans. Am. Neurol. Assoc.,* 95:259–261.
60. Heilman, K. M., Pandya, D. N., Karol, E. A., and Geschwind, N. (1971): Auditory inattention. *Arch. Neurol.,* 24:323–325.
61. Heilman, K. M., and Valenstein, E. (1972): Auditory neglect in man. *Arch. Neurol.,* 26:32–35.
62. Heilman, K. M., and Valenstein, E. (1972): Frontal lobe neglect in man. *Neurology (Minneap.),* 22:660–664.
63. Holmes, G. (1918): Disturbances of visual orientation. *Br. J. Ophthalmol.,* 2:449–506.
64. Holmes, G. (1919): Disturbances of visual space perception. *Br. Med. J.,* 2:230–233.
65. Holmes, G. and Horrax, G. (1919): Disturbances of spatial orientation and visual attention, with loss of stereoscopic vision. *Arch. Neurol. Psychiatry,* 1:385–407.
66. Jackson, J. H. (1876): Case of large cerebral tumour without optic neuritis and with left hemiplegia and imperception. In: *Selected Writings of John Hughlings Jackson,* edited by James Taylor, pp. 146–152. Hodden and Stoughton, London (1932).
67. Juba, A. (1949): Beitrag zur Struktur dev ein-und doppelseitigen körper-schemastövemgen Fingeragnosie, atypische Anosognosien. *Mschr. Psychiat. Neurol.,* 118:11–29. [Quoted by Critchley, M. (1953): *The Parietal Lobes,* Hafner, New York.]
68. Kanareikin, K. F., Babenkova, S. V., and Romel, T. E. (1976): Mental changes in local vascular lesions of right hemisphere. In: *Cerebral Vascular Diseases, Seventh International Conference, Salzburg,* edited by J. S. Meyer, H. Lechner, and M. Reivich, pp. 106–108. Thieme Pub., Stuttgart.
69. Kennard, M. A. (1939): Alterations in response to visual stimuli following lesions of frontal lobe in monkeys. *Arch. Neurol. Psychiatry,* 41:1153–1165.
70. Kimura, D. (1973): The asymmetry of the human brain. In: *Recent Progress in Perception,* pp. 246–254. W. H. Freeman and Co., San Francisco.
71. Kinsbourne, M., and Warrington, E. (1963): Jargon aphasia. *Neuropsychologia,* 1:27–37.
72. Kinsbourne, M. (1974): Direction of gaze and distribution of cerebral thought processes. *Neuropsychologia,* 12:279–281.
73. Kimura, D. (1964): Left–right differences in the perception of melodies. *Q. J. Exp. Psychol.,* 16:355–358.
74. Kinsbourne, M. (1970): A model for the mechanism of unilateral neglect of space. *Trans. Am. Neurol. Assoc.,* 95:143–146.
75. Kirvel, R. D. (1975): Sensorimotor responsiveness in rats with unilateral superior collicular and amygdaloid lesions. *J. Comp. Physiol. Psychol.,* 8:882–891.
76. Kirvel, R. D., Greenfield, R. A., and Meyer, D. R. (1974): Multimodal sensory neglect in rats with radical unilateral posterior isocortical and superior collicular ablations. *J. Comp. Physiol. Psychol.,* 87:156–162.
77. Kleist, K. (1912): Der gang und der gegenivärtige Stand der Apraxieforschung. *Ergehn. Neurol. Psychiat.,* 1:342–452. [Quoted by Benson, D. F., and Barton, M. I. (1970): Disturbances in constructional ability. *Cortex,* 6:19–46.]
78. Kleist, K. (1922): In: *Handbuch der arztlichen Erfahrungen in Weltkriege,* 4:343. [Quoted by Brain, W. R. (1941): Visual disorientation with special reference to lesions of the right cerebral hemisphere. *Brain,* 64:244–272.]
79. Kleist, K. (1934): *Gehirnpathologie.* Barth, Liepzig.

80. Kleist, K. (1934): Konstruktive (optische) apraxie. In: *Handbuch der artzlichen Erfahrungen in Weltkriege 1914/1918,* edited by K. Bonhoeffer. Barth, Liepzig. [Quoted by Benson, D. F., and Barton, M. I. (1970): Disturbances in constructional ability. *Cortex,* 6:19–46.]

81. Lhermitte, J., and de Ajuriaguerra, J. (1942): *Psychopathologie de la vision.* Masson, Paris.

82. McFie, J., Piercy, M. F., and Zangwill, O. L. (1950): Visual–spatial agnosia associated with lesions of the right cerebral hemisphere. *Brain,* 73:167–190.

83. McFie, J., and Zangwill, O. L. (1960): Visual constructive disabilities associated with lesions of the left cerebral hemisphere. *Brain,* 83:243–260.

84. Marie, P. (1918): In discussion of paper by Babinski, J. (1918): Anosognosie. *Rev. Neurol. (Paris),* 25:365–367.

85. Marie, P., Bouttier, H., and Bailey, P. (1922): La planotopokinésie, étude sur les erreurs d'exécution de certains mouvements dans leurs rapports avec la représentation spatiale. *Rev. Neurol. (Paris),* I:505–512.

86. Marshall, J. F., Turner, B. H., and Teitelbaum, P. (1971): Sensory neglect produced by lateral hypothalamic damage. *Science,* 174:523–525.

87. Milner, B. and Taylor, T. (1972): Right hemisphere superiority in tactile pattern recognition after cerebral commissurotomy: Evidence of nonverbal memory. *Neuropsychologia,* 10:1–15.

88. Milner, B., Taylor, L., and Sperry, R. W. (1968): Lateralized suppression of dichotically presented digits after commissural section in man. *Science,* 161:184–186.

89. Mountcastle, V. B. (1975): *The World Around Us: Neural Command Functions for Selective Attention.* The F. O. Schmitt Lecture in Neuroscience. Neurosciences research program.

90. Mountcastle, V. B. (1976): F. O. Schmitt Lecture in Neuroscience. Neurosciences research program, bulletin 15, supplement.

91. Nielsen, J. M. (1938): Disturbances of the body scheme. *Bull. Los Angeles Neurol. Soc.,* 3:127–135.

92. Nielsen, J. M. (1938): Gerstmann syndrome, finger agnosia, agraphia, confusion of right and left and acalculia. *Arch. Neurol. Psychiatry,* 39:536–590.

93. Obersteiner, H. (1881): On allochiria, a peculiar sensory disorder. *Brain,* 4:153–163.

94. Oppenheim, H. (1885): Ueber eine durch eine klinisch bisher nicht verwertete Untersuchungsmethode ermittelte Form der Sensibilitatsstorung bei einseitigen Erkrankungen des Grosshirns (Kurze Mitteilung). *Neurol. Centrabl.,* 23:529–533.

95. Oxbury, J. M., Campbell, D. C., and Oxbury, S. M. (1974): Unilateral spatial neglect. *Brain,* 97:551–564.

96. Paterson, A., and Zangwill, O. L. (1944): Disorders of visual space perception associated with lesions of the right cerebral hemisphere. *Brain,* 67:331–358.

97. Paterson, A., and Zangwill, O. L. (1945): A case of topographical disorientation associated with a unilateral cerebral lesion. *Brain,* 68:188–212.

98. Pick, A. (1898): Quoted by Gerstmann, J. (1942): Problem of imperception of disease and of impaired body territories with organic lesions. *Arch. Neurol. Psychiatry,* 48:890–913.

99. Pick, A. (1903): On reduplicative paramnesia. *Brain,* 26:260–267.

100. Pick, A. (1908): *Ueber Störungen der Orientierung am eigenen Körper in Arbeiten aus der Psychiatrischen. Klin. Prag.* I, Berlin, Karger.

101. Pick, A. (1922): Störung der orientierung am eigenen Körper. *Psychol. Forsch.,* I:303–318.

102. Pinéas, H. (1926): Der mangel an Krankheitsbewusstein und seine variationen als symptom organische Erkrankungen. *Verh. Dtsch. Ges. Deseh. Nervenarzte,* 16:238–248.

103. Pinéas, H. (1931): Ein Fall von räumilichen Orientierungsstörung mit Dyschirie. *Z. Ges. Neurol. Psychiat.,* 113:180–195.

104. Poppelreuter, W. K. (1917): *Die psychischen Schadigungen durch Kopfschuss im Krieg 1914–1916: Die Störungen der niederen und höheren Leistungen durch Verletzungen des Okzipitalhirns.* Vol. 1. Leopold Voss, Leipzig.

105. Pötzl, O. (1928): *Die Aphasialehre vom Standpunkte der klinischen Psychiatrie. Bd. 1, Die optisch—agnostischen Störungen.* Leipzig. [Quoted by Brain, W. R. (1941): Visual disorientation with special reference to lesions of the right cerebral hemisphere. *Brain,* 64:244–272.]

106. Redlich, E., and Bonvicini, G. (1908): Ueber das Fehlen der Wahrnehmung der eigeney Blindkeit bei Hirnkrankheiten. *Jahrbl. Psychiatr.,* 29:1–134.

107. Reeves, A. J., and Hagamen, W. D. (1971): Behavioral and EEG asymmetry following unilateral lesions of the forebrain and midbrain of ctas. *Electroencephalogr. Clin. Neurophysiol.,* 30:83–86.

108. Riddoch, G. (1935): Visual disorientation in homonymous half-fields. *Brain,* 58:376–382.

109. Reider, N. (1946): Phenomena of sensory suppression. *Arch. Neurol. Psychiatry,* 55:583–590.
110. Roth, M. (1949): Disorders of the body image caused by lesions of the right parietal lobe. *Brain,* 72:89–111.
111. Rubens, A. B., Mahowald, M. W., and Hutton, J. T. (1976): Asymmetry of the lateral (sylvian) fissures in man. *Neurology (Minneap.),* 26:620–624.
112. Rudel, R. G., Denckla, M. B., and Spalten, E. (1974): The functional asymmetry of Braille letter learning in normal sighted children. *Neurology (Minneap.),* 24:733–738.
113. Sandifer, P. H. (1946): Anosognosia and disorders of body scheme. *Brain,* 69:122–137.
114. Scheller, H., and Seidemann, H. (1931): Zur Frage der Optischraumlichen Agnosie (zugleich ein Beitrag zur Dyslexie). *Mschr. Psychiat. Neurol.,* 81:97–188. [Quoted by Critchley, M. (1953): *The Parietal Lobes,* Hafner, New York.]
115. Schilder, P. (1932): Localization of the body image (postural model of the body). *Ass. Res. Nerv. Ment. Dis.,* 13:466–484.
116. Schilder, P. (1935): *The Image and Appearance of the Human Body.* Kegan Paul, Trench, Trubner, and Co., London.
117. Schilder, P., and Stengel, E. (1928): Schmerzasymbolie. *Z. Ges. Neurol. Psychiat.,* 113:143.
118. Schwartz, G. E., Davidson, R. J., and Maer, F. (1975): Right hemisphere lateralization for emotion in the human brain: Interactions with cognition. *Science,* 190:286–288.
119. Semmes, J., Weinstein, S., Ghent, L., and Teuber, H. L. (1960): *Somatosensory Changes after Penetrating Brain Wounds in Man.* Harvard University Press, Cambridge.
120. Shapiro, M. F., Fink, M., and Bender, M. B. (1952): Exosomesthesia or displacement of cutaneous sensation into extrapersonal space. *Arch. Neurol. Psychiatry,* 68:481–490.
121. Silberpfennig, J. (1941): Contribution to the problem of eye movements. III. Disturbances of ocular movements with pseudohemianopia in frontal lobe tumors. *Confin. Neurol.,* 4:1–13.
122. Smith, A. (1972): *Dominant and Non-Dominant Hemispherectomy in Drugs, Development and Cerebral Function,* edited by W. L. Smith. Charles C Thomas, Springfield, Ill.
123. Spellacy, F., and Blumstein, S. (1970): The influence of language set and ear preference in phoneme recognition. *Cortex,* 6:430–439.
124. Sperry, R. W. (1974): Lateral specialization in the surgically separated hemispheres. In: *The Neurosciences, Third Study Program,* edited by F. O. Schmitt and F. G. Warden, pp. 5–21. MIT Press, Cambridge.
125. Sprague, J. M. (1966): Interaction of cortex and superior colliculus in mediation of visually guided behavior in the cat. *Science,* 153:1544–1547.
126. Sprague, J. M., Chambers, W. W., and Stellar, E. (1961): Attentive, affective and adaptive behavior in the cat. *Science,* 133:165–173.
127. Sprague, J. M., and Meikle, T. H. (1965): The role of the superior colliculus in visually guided behavior. *Exp. Neurol.,* 11:115–146.
128. Teng, E. L., and Sperry, R. W. (1974): Interhemispheric rivalry during simultaneous bilateral task presentation in commissurotomized patients. *Cortex,* 10:111–120.
129. Thiebaut, F., and Guillaumet, L. (1945): Hemianopsie relative. *Rev. Neurol. (Paris),* 77:129.
130. Trevarthen, C. (1974): *Personal communication.*
131. Ungerstedt, U. (1973): Selective lesions of central catecholamine pathways: Application in functional studies. In: *Neurosciences Research,* edited by S. Ehrenpreis and I. Kopin, pp. 73–96. Academic Press, New York.
132. Ungerstedt, U. (1974): Brain dopamine neurons and behavior. In: *The Neurosciences. Third Study Program,* edited by F. O. Schmitt and F. G. Worden, pp. 695–703. MIT Press, Cambridge.
133. Vercelli, G. (1947): Interesse e significato de fenomeno della eclissi della sensibilita in una meta del corpo al doppio stimolo simultaneo e simmetrico in determinate sinformi da lesione dell emisfero cerebrale opposto. *Rev. Neurol.,* 17:243–252. [Quoted by Bender, M. B. (1952): *Disorders in Perception.* Charles C Thomas, Springfield, Ill.]
134. Von Monakow, C. (1885): Experimentelle und pathologisch–anatomische Untersuchungen über die Beziehungen der sogenannten Sehsphare zu den infrakortikalen Opticuscentren und zum N. opticus. *Arch. Psychiatr.,* 16:151–371.
135. Wada, J. A., Clarke, R., and Hamm, A. (1975): Cerebral hemispheric asymmetry in humans: Cortical speech zones in 100 adult and 100 infant brains. *Arch. Neurol.,* 32:239–246.
136. Warrington, E. K. (1962): Completion of visual forms across hemianopic field defects. *J. Neurol. Neurosurg. Psychiatry,* 25:208.
137. Watson, R. T., Heilman, K. M., Cauthen, J. C., and King, F. A. (1973): Neglect after cingulectomy. *Neurology (Minneap.),* 23:1003–1007.

138. Watson, R. T., Heilman, K. M., Miller, B. D., and King, F. A. (1974): Neglect after mesence-phalic reticular formation lesions. *Neurology (Minneap.)*, 24:294–298.
139. Weinstein, E. A. (1976): The use of sodium amytal for testing mental function. *J. Mt. Sinai Hosp.*, 33:269–277.
140. Weinstein, E. A., and Cole, M. (1963): Concepts of anosognosia. In: *Problems of Dynamic Neurology*, edited by L. Halpern. Jerusalem Post Press, Jerusalem.
141. Weinstein, E. A., Cole, M., Mitchell, M. S., and Lyerly, O. (1964): Anosognosia and aphasia. *Arch. Neurol. Psychiatry*, 10:376–386.
142. Weinstein, E. A., Lyerly, O. G., Cole, M., and Ozer, M. N. (1966): Meaning in jargon aphasia. *Cortex*, 2:165–187.
143. Weinstein, E. A., and Kahn, R. L. (1952): Non-aphasic misnaming (paraphasia) in organic brain disease. *Arch. Neurol. Psychiatry*, 67:72–79.
144. Weinstein, E. A., and Kahn, R. L. (1955): *Denial of Illness*. Charles C Thomas, Springfield, Ill.
145. Weinstein, E. A., and Kahn, R. L. (1961): Patterns of sexual behavior following brain injury. *Psychiatry*, 24:69–78.
146. Weinstein, E. A., Kahn, R. L., and Slote, W. H. (1955): Withdrawal, inattention and pain asymbolia. *Arch. Neurol. Psychiatry*, 74:235–248.
147. Weinstein, E. A., Kahn, R. L., and Sugarman, L. A. (1954): Ludic behavior in patients with brain disease. *J. Hillside Hosp.*, 3:98–106.
148. Weinstein, E. A., and Lyerly, O. G. (1968): Confabulation following brain injury. *Arch. Gen. Psychiatry*, 18:348–354.
149. Welch, K., and Stuteville, P. (1958): Experimental production of unilateral neglect in monkeys. *Brain*, 81:341–347.
150. Wilbrand, H. (1892): *Dtsch. Z. Nervenheilk.*, 2:361. [Quoted by Brain, W. R. (1941): Visual disorientation with special references to lesions of the right cerebral hemisphere. *Brain*, 64: 244–272.]
151. Zaidel, E. (1974): Language, dichotic listening and the disconnected hemispheres. Paper presented at the *Conference on Human Brain Function*, UCLA, September 27, 1974.
152. Zaidel, E. (1975): The case of the elusive right hemisphere. Paper presented at the *13th Annual Meeting of the Academy of Aphasia*, Victoria, B.C., October 7, 1975.
153. Zaidel, E. (1977): Laterality effects with the token test. *Neuropsychologia. (In press.)*
154. Zaidel, E. (1977): Auditory vocabulary of the right hemisphere following brain bisection or hemi-decortication. *Cortex. (In press.)*
155. Zangwill, O. L. (1963): The completion effect in hemianopia and its relation to anosognosia. In: *Problems of Dynamic Neurology*, edited by L. Halpern. Jerusalem Post Press, Jerusalem.
156. Zarit, S. H., and Kahn, R. L. (1974): Impairment and adaptation in chronic disabilities: Spatial inattention. *J. Nerv. Ment. Dis.*, 159:63–72.
157. Zingerle, H. (1913): Ueber Störungen der Wahrnehmung des eigenen Körpers bei organischen Gehirnerkrankungen. *Mschr. Psychiatr. Neurol.*, 34:13–36.

Advances in Neurology, Vol. 18, edited by E. A.
Weinstein and R. P. Friedland. Raven Press,
New York © 1977.

Inattention Syndromes in Split-Brain Man

Robert J. Joynt

*Department of Neurology, University of Rochester Medical Center,
Rochester, New York 14642*

Attention is a mental state much like consciousness, which, William James noted, was understood by everyone until attempts were made to define it. Kimura and Durnford (8) note ". . . a term such as 'attention' is so vague as to be of little use in understanding the details of how the left and right hemisphere actually operate." In this chapter, I use the term attention to mean the ordering of our mental processes to note information so that it can subsequently be processed, and, in some instances, acted on. This assumes that the peripheral mechanisms for bringing that information into the central nervous system are intact. The breakdown of this orderly concatenation we can call inattention. By clinical testing, this is arrived at by noting the patient does not respond properly to some stimulus—the complexity of the proferred stimulus and expected response can vary from a simple movement to complex behavior. In many instances, we cannot discern where the system falls apart. Occasionally, we have the impression that the individual perceives the information but cannot process it or act on it, but there is no absolute proof that the patient attended to the stimulus at the onset. This definition of "inattention" is not totally satisfactory. It might include the agnosias, apraxias, and aphasias. But if we can, through any modality, be certain the patient was aware of the stimulus, then we can eliminate inattention as the break in the chain and speculate about some other disorder. It is a particular problem when we examine split-brain man, for here we have separated for some mental tasks the sensory input center from the processing center or, perhaps, these two from the effector. Therefore, the patient may fail our clinical test and we might erroneously assume unawareness or inattention.

Examples of this dilemma are not common. A recent instance was in a patient I observed who suffered from a right anterior cerebral artery infarction with little motor or sensory deficit in the left arm. The patient reported an unusual occurrence, which was repeated on several occasions. When seated at a table and writing out checks with the right hand, the left hand would gently rise up, grasp the right hand, and move it aside. All of this was a complete surprise to the patient and only when the right hand was forcibly moved did he attend to actions of the left. The action of the left hand was not the common levitation phenomenon seen with parietal sensory loss but a purposeful and directed movement. The speculation was an anterior callosal deconnection with independently reacting hemispheres. The problem arises as to whether or not there was inattention to the actions of the left hand. The patient verbally disavowed awareness when asked, indicating that his left hemisphere was inattentive. Is it proper to assume the right hemisphere was equally ignorant? This was a complicated motor act. One does not have to be very analytical to recognize the teleological significance of this behavior. Yet I cannot indict the right hemisphere; it sits there mute and its culpability is not established.

Many other examples of this peculiar behavior have been noted. Akelaitis and his colleagues (1) used the term diagonistic dyspraxia. They relate cases of post-commissurotomy patients who opened drawers with one hand while closing them with the other or dressed with one hand and undressed with the other.

When the behavior of post-commissurotomy patients is examined in detail, many other examples of inattention are revealed. In the laboratory situation, it is easier to analyze this behavior and often demonstrate that inattention is not, in fact, the problem. Examples of this are well known but a few reports will illustrate the point. Tachistoscopic presentation of object pictures or written material to the left half-field will usually not produce a correct identifying response and the patient will deny knowledge of the presentation. At this point we could conclude that split-brain patients have an inattention syndrome affecting the left field of vision. However, the patient can with his left hand pick out and match the object to its picture and can often match some objects to written material. Similar experiments utilizing various inputs and outputs can identify other so-called inattention syndromes that evaporate when the response can be wrested from the brain by using other modalities. Most of the apparent inattention syndromes in split-brain man are manifested by the inability to give a verbal answer or a correct verbal answer to a stimulus presentation to the right hemisphere. Interestingly, if an answer is given and it is false, the mute but not deaf right side will register its disgust and frustration by appropriate facial grimacing (14), again confirming that lack of awareness or inattention is not the problem.

Why inattention syndromes are not encountered more frequently in these split-brain patients in day-to-day behavior or in laboratory testing is a puzzle. But why should we expect inattention syndromes? First, numerous studies have confirmed the importance of the commissures in transferring information from one side of the brain to the other. Second, there is the notion voiced by Eccles (2) that the right hemisphere is devoid of consciousness. Certainly then, with the split-brain, it seems we have the proper conditions to have or appear to have many varieties of inattention syndromes.

An argument for the scarcity of inattention states is the ability of the brain to compensate after a time. This is likely not an explanation in many cases. This notion has been put forth for the lack of enduring disturbances in callosal sectioned patients. If there is compensation, it is not complete, as deficits in transfer of information still remain after 30 years in two of the patients reported by Akelaitis and his colleagues in the early 1940s. These were manifest with defects in transfer of learning with simple hand sorting and placement tasks and in crossed intermodal identification. In spite of these defects, there were no reports by these patients of behavior that could be called inattention defects (5,6).

Another reason why splitting the brain may have few consequences is the redundancy of the sensory input systems so that eliminating transcallosal transmission hinders, but does not definitely disrupt, some information gathering pathways. The redundancy and distribution of these systems vary in individuals, which may account for the behavioral differences noted after presumably similar commissurotomies or in patients with agenesis of the corpus callosum. At an experimental level, this variation can be studied in normal, commissurotomized and callosal agenesis subjects with cortical evoked potentials. The relative contribution of ipsilateral and contralateral sensory pathways can be noted (7). The discrepancy in the relative contribution can be quite marked, with some having excellent ipsilateral sensory input in spite of no transcallosal contribution. Therefore, the amount of information getting to the ipsilateral and presumably isolateral hemispheres may not be greatly diminished (Fig. 1).

Furthermore, inattention syndromes occur less frequently in split-brain patients than in those with focal cerebral lesions. Kinsbourne (11) points out that areas of the brain inhibit other areas potentially capable of that function. He cites several clinical examples, such as the emergence of right-hemisphere speech

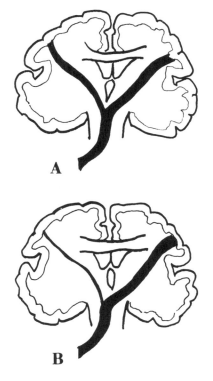

A

B

FIG. 1. Possible differences in the sensory input systems with varying contributions of the ipsilateral pathways. Commissurotomy would affect the "isolated hemisphere" more in B than in A.

function after left-hemisphere damage. Thus, commissurotomy would disinhibit certain areas so that the separated hemispheres would, in fact, be less vulnerable to inattention behavior. It has been shown that disconnected hemispheres are more efficient at processing certain information than is the united brain (3).

A further reason for the lack of findings is the possible utilization of a dual sensory and motor system (15). In experimental animals, including primates, there is an infracortical visual and motor system that is unaffected by commissurotomy. In the visual sphere, animals can localize and orient attention to objects when the visual cortex has been ablated. Similar findings are present in motor systems so that there is an infracortical system regulating the gross movement of the hand. Precise manipulation is a cortical function. These systems likely account, in part, for the relatively normal attention and behavior observed in split-brain man, for much of our ongoing behavior is relatively casual and does not require a high degree of visual scrutiny or motor manipulation. It is only when we push these systems to the limit, as in our artificial testing procedures, that defects can be demonstrated.

Lastly, it is essential to examine the expressed notion that the right hemisphere in post-commissurotomy patients does not possess consciousness. For without consciousness there can be no attention. Eccles (2) states, ". . . . the conscious self, with all its linguistic and sophisticated behavioral performance, seems to be represented solely in the dominant hemisphere in these split-brain patients." As evidence, Eccles points out the inability to assign consciousness to the right hemisphere in the absence of symbolic communication. This idea is gainsaid by several observations. It is apparent to other examiners and to myself when examining these patients that the right hemisphere can tell when the left hemisphere gives a false answer and, although lacking the ability to admonish verbally, can, by appropriate facial expressions and head shaking, express disagreement—evidence that I would accept beyond peradventure as awareness and a conscious effort of expression, although not employing verbal symbols. In fact, the right hemisphere does have language capabilities and it has been amply demonstrated that, with damage to the left hemisphere, it is the right hemisphere that is responsible for the residual speech (9,13). As further evidence for his idea, Eccles also notes that the right hemisphere is not capable of volitional movements on its own. However, the separated right hemisphere is perfectly capable of independent volitional control. For example, these patients can imitate, with both hands, pictures of hand and finger positions shown to the left half-field, so that only the right hemisphere possessed the knowledge to initiate the motor act (4).

For all of these reasons, inattention defects are not common in split-brain patients. What role, then, does the corpus callosum play in attention? The two hemispheres have disparate functions, as shown by many lines of evidence. It is likely from the study of fetal brains that the hemispheres are preprogrammed this way (16). It is also likely from the study of infantile hemiplegia that one hemisphere cannot totally take over the functions of the other (17). Thus, each half brain is equipped with unique properties. However, it is rare that any complex behavior requires only the attention of one to the exclusion of the other hemisphere. It is difficult to envision any complicated behavior that could not profitably draw on the talents of both hemispheres. Kinsbourne (10) points out that one of the biologically significant functions of the corpus callosum is the equalizing of hemispheric function so that it minimizes the disparities in the distribution of mental capacity or attention. Therefore, both can be rapidly involved in any activity in which bilateral involvement is beneficial. He and his colleagues also point out that, in split-brain patients, when this attention cannot be distributed, one hemisphere can be overloaded if it has too much to do (12). This was illustrated by having normal subjects and a split-brain patient tap their fingers when talking. When the split-brain patient was groping for a verbal response, tapping ceased with the right hand, whereas it did not in the normals. They interpreted this as the inability of the separated left hemisphere to draw on the resources of the other when the store of attention was depleted in the effort to find a verbal response.

In summary, inattention syndromes are encountered in split-brain man, but they are uncommon and many are partial. The reasons for the relative infrequency are not because of the ability of the brain to compensate but because of the redundancy of the information systems, the disinhibition of the separated hemisphere, the employment of alternative sensory and motor systems, and the persisting consciousness or awareness in both separated hemispheres. The role of the corpus callosum is to minimize the disparities in the distribution of mental capacity and attention so that the function of both hemispheres can be utilized in appropriate and effective behavior.

ACKNOWLEDGMENTS

This work was supported by Grant No. 05084 NINCDS, National Institutes of Health and The Waasdorp Fund for Stroke Research.

REFERENCES

1. Akelaitis, A. J., Risteen, W. A., Herren, R. Y., and Van Wagenen, W. P. (1952): Studies on the corpus callosum. III. A contribution to the study of dyspraxia and apraxia following partial and complete section of the corpus callosum. *Arch. Neurol. Psychiatry,* 47:971–1008.
2. Eccles, J. C. (1965): *The Brain and Unity of Conscious Experience.* Eddington Memorial Lecture, Cambridge University Press, Cambridge, England.
3. Gazzaniga, M. S. (1968): Short-term memory and brain-bisected man. *Psychonom. Sci.,* 12: 161–163.
4. Gazzaniga, M. S., Bogen, J. E., and Sperry, R. W. (1967): Dyspraxia following division of the cerebral commissures. *Arch. Neurol.,* 12:606–612.
5. Goldstein, M. N., and Joynt, R. J. (1969): Long term follow-up of a callosal sectioned patient. *Arch. Neurol.,* 20:96–102.
6. Goldstein, M. N., Joynt, R. J., and Hartley, R. (1975): Long-term effects of callosal sectioning. *Arch. Neurol.,* 32:52–54.
7. Joynt, R. J., and McAdam, D.: *(Unpublished observations.)*
8. Kimura, D., and Durnford, M. (1974): Normal studies on the right hemisphere in vision. In:

Hemisphere Function in the Human Brain, edited by S. J. Dimond and J. G. Beaumont. Wiley and Sons, New York.

9. Kinsbourne, M. (1971): The minor cerebral hemisphere as a source of aphasic speech. *Arch. Neurol.,* 25:302–306.
10. Kinsbourne, M. (1974): Lateral interactions in the brain. In: *Hemispheric Disconnection and Cerebral Function,* edited by M. Kinsbourne and W. L. Smith. Charles C Thomas, Springfield, Ill.
11. Kinsbourne, M. (1974): Mechanisms of hemispheric interaction in man. In: *Hemispheric Disconnection and Cerebral Function,* edited by M. Kinsbourne and W. L. Smith. Charles C Thomas, Springfield, Ill.
12. Kreuter, C., Kinsbourne, M., and Trevarthen, C. (1972): Are disconnected cerebral hemispheres independent channels? A preliminary study of the effect of unilateral loading on bilateral finger tapping. *Neuropsychologia,* 10:453–461.
13. Mempel, E., Svebrzynska, J., Sobczynska, J., and Zarski, S. (1963): Compensation of speech disorders by nondominant cerebral hemisphere in adults. J. Neurol. Neurosurg. Psychiatry, 26:96.
14. Sperry, R. W. (1968): Hemisphere disconnection and unity in conscious awareness. *Am. Psychol.,* 23:723–733.
15. Trevarthen, C. (1974): Functional relations of disconnected hemispheres with the brain stem and with each other: Monkey and man. In: *Hemispheric Disconnection and Cerebral Function,* edited by M. Kinsbourne and W. L. Smith. Charles C Thomas, Springfield, Ill.
16. Witelson, S. F., and Pallie, W. (1973): Left-hemisphere specialization for language in the human newborn: Neuroanatomical evidence of asymmetry. *Brain,* 96:641–646.
17. Woods, B. T., and Teuber, H. L. (1973): Early onset of complementary specialization of cerebral hemispheres in man. *Trans. Am. Neurol. Assoc.,* 98:113–117.

DISCUSSION

Dr. Heilman: Can I ask a question of Dr. Joynt? Has anybody looked at neglect, unilateral neglect, using verbal versus nonverbal simultaneous stimulation, meaning you say to the patient, "I'm going to touch you on the right, left, or both, and you tell me right, left, or both," and the other condition being "I'm going to touch you right, left, or both, and if I touch your right hand raise your right hand; if I touch your left hand raise your left hand; if I touch both hands raise both hands." What do you expect from lesions both of the corpus callosum and the right parietal lobe, and what would they do with these tasks? Has it been done?

Dr. Joynt: I would guess the split-brain patient would be able to perform under both conditions—the tasks are simple and there are too many opportunities for cross-cueing. The problem with a right parietal lesion is more complex, as the sensory information from the left side may be inadequate with cortical sensory loss, extinction, etc. Each condition is the same as far as touching and performing the same motoric task, except for one: you're not asking him to lift but are asking for a complete verbal response, and, in the other one, you're asking each hemisphere to do its own thing. In other words, one needs a corpus callosum and the other hypothetically doesn't.

Dr. Weinstein: Dr. Joynt has given us some crucial information. He notes that the clinical manifestations of hemi-inattention following callosal section are inconspicuous, and he attributes this to the use of other information systems that do not travel across the corpus callosum. The right hemisphere does "know" a good deal of what is going on, or what is not going on, in the left field of space and the body, although, like an aphasic patient, it cannot name the object specifically. However, as Dr. Joynt has pointed out, it may use emotional language and gesture, and, in this sense, the right hemisphere is both "conscious" and "attentive." The preservation of consciousness is in accordance with the intactness of the connections between the two sides of the brain through the brainstem and the hypothalamic commissures.

In the patient with conspicuous hemi-inattention associated with neoplastic invasion, infarcts, and direct trauma to a hemisphere, there is involvement of the limbic reticular system and an impairment of consciousness. We might, then, call hemi-inattention, hemi-consciousness, if you will forgive the neologism. The patient "knows" in some ways about the affected side, but acts and talks as if it were not there. He expresses this knowledge in "emotional" language, in gesture, metaphor, and personification. That there are specific pathways for "emotional" information we know from the experiments of Mountcastle. Here we have a nice distinction between the neurological definition of consciousness as awareness and the psychological usage of the term to indicate knowledge in a referential context of an event or experience, but lack of awareness of the processes of selective perception and emotional set that determine idiosyncratic or experiential meaning.

At this point we might consider the effects of other iatrogenic lesions. I refer to ablations of the parietal cortex done for scarring and the relief of pain, and to hemispherectomy. These results, of course, have to be approached cautiously because of the existence of prior brain damage. In a series of right parietal cortical ablations performed by Dr. Wilder Penfield and studied by Henry Hecaen, all six subjects had contralateral extinction, but the more conspicuous manifestations of hemi-neglect, beyond the immediate postoperative period, were meager. Similarly, Aaron Smith, from his experience with hemispherectomy, has found extinction but not the more severe verbal and nonverbal signs of hemi-inattention. My guess is that in order for the existence of conspicuous multimodal and intermodal hemi-neglect, we need not only a hemisphere imbalance but a disturbance in corticolimbic reticular activation that does not occur after either cortical ablation or hemispherectomy. That some active process is involved is suggested by the fact that hemi-inattention is most apt to develop with rapidly occurring or developing lesions and that it subsides when the lesions are quiescent. In support, I can cite the similarities between full blown hemi-inattention and the amnestic-confabulatory state, in which the confabulations often disappear in time.

Advances in Neurology, Vol. 18, edited by E. A. Weinstein and R. P. Friedland. Raven Press, New York © 1977.

Hemi-Neglect and Hemisphere Rivalry

Marcel Kinsbourne

Neuropsychology Research Unit, The Hospital for Sick Children, Toronto, Ontario, Canada M5G IX8

In this chapter I will use the subject of unilateral neglect as a vehicle for discussing the organization of right- and left-orienting tendencies and their relationship to lateralized cognitive function. My presentation is directed toward the level of behavior.

In what Pasik might describe as a classical counter-Benderian tradition, I will begin with my models and then present some circumstantial evidence in favor of them. There are control centers in the brain for rightward and for leftward orientation, which are in mutually inhibitory interaction (7). By rightward orientation, I mean turning of the body, head, and eyes to the right; turning of the head and eyes right; turning of the eyes right; or merely a submotor shift of attention with maintained central fixation. All will be attributed to the same mechanism (and vice versa for leftward orientation).

Although these are opposing influences, they are not necessarily equal and opposite influences. In the human, for example, the rightward-orienting tendency subserved by the left half brain is more powerful. I will discuss what happens to this reciprocal balance when one or the other control mechanism is selectively inactivated or stimulated. Finally, I will consider the evidence that on each side the lateralized cognitive processes (verbal on the left and spatial on the right) interact, in terms of level of activation, with the lateral orientor of the same side, and I will argue that neglect is based on a selective incapacity of one of the two lateral orienting systems. I will not commit myself to a neuroanatomical level because a single phenomenon can occur at various levels. The clinical phenomenon of unilateral neglect represents such an imbalance, and the asymmetry in incidence and the greater severity of left-sided neglect (1) are to be explained either by this asymmetry in initial leftward and rightward tendencies or by interactions between processor and orientor on each side, or in both of these ways. What I am attempting to provide is a heuristic framework for a number of miscellaneous observations that will lead up to a plausible thesis.

Let me start by making the case for hemi-inattention being an imbalance in the lateral orienting tendency. Clinically, it is obvious that neglect phenomena are different than the phenomena of sensory loss in any individual sensory modality. For instance, take a variant on the usual way of testing for the extinction of one of two simultaneous visual presentations. If we test this not by putting one stimulus on either side of the patient's midline but by putting both into his intact half field of vision, we find that the patient attends to the more lateral of the two horizontally adjacent stimuli. This demonstrates a lateral orienting to the more eccentric of the stimuli, as predicted by imbalance in the "seesaw" mechanism proposed. If one of the two control mechanisms is out of kilter, the other swings to the outside as far as the stimulus permits. Another everyday clinical observation in patients with neglect can be made by having the patient close his eyes while you put a newspaper in front of him. You then say to him "open your eyes and read this paper." You can watch him open his eyes and turn them all the way across, very quickly, to the outer margin of the sheet (apparently oblivious of what he is doing). Irrespective of where you hold the paper, he will go to the lateral border of the print on the page. The point is that the orienting will be to the end of the structured visual field, ipsilateral to the lesion, wherever it may be. The bias is not with reference to any particular locus in the visual field, but to one end of a laterally extended display, regardless of where that is located.

Gross neglect is an acute phenomenon that rarely lasts for a long period of time after onset. Some years ago, in England, I worked with a series of 130 veterans who had sustained penetrating missile wounds of the head in combat in Normandy 20 years earlier (2). Not one of these patients had neglect in any way that a neurologist could recognize it. However, on tachistoscopy, some suggestive findings appeared. Sets of four letters at a time were flashed in one of two ways. Either they were horizontally aligned, two in each visual field, or there was a rectangular block of four in the intact visual field ipsilateral to the lesion. We scored errors and also looked at the serial position effect on accuracy. With bilateral presentation, the patients with left lesions did better on the left end of the stimulus, as do normals. The patients with right-hemisphere lesions actually had the opposite serial position curve. They did better with the rightmost letters, consistent with a right-to-left scan, a reversed direction of scan of the rapidly fading visual trace.

Even more flagrantly, the results of the unilateral rectangular displays showed that the patients with left-hemisphere lesions did better on the leftmost pair (vertically adjacent), and the patients with right-hemisphere lesions did best on the rightmost pair, even when all four letters were in the intact visual field (ipsilateral to the lesion). So, clearly, it is the relative position in lateral space that is the determinant of what is ignored and what is not ignored, rather than the absolute locus in one or the other half field or in some part of the half field.

The corollary of inadequate exploration to one side is exaggerated exploration of the other side. There is a phantasmagoria of clinical observations suggesting that patients with left-sided neglect are overresponsive to and, as it were, magnetically attracted by the rightmost extremity of display, even when this does not seem to have much adaptive significance. There is a wealth of information from animal species at various levels of evolution suggesting that these lateral balances in right- and left-orienting tendencies are a very ancient and primitive arrangement, characterizing not only the human species but even the simplest existing bisymmetrical freely moving organism (7). We are not dealing with some exclusive arrangement for looking right and left, but with the programming of a basic animal behavior without which the species could not survive—the ability to orient to the right, to the left, for adaptive purposes, toward food, predators, and so on (10).

The balance is not necessarily equal and opposite. I am not saying that rightward orienting tendencies are overridingly more potent, but rather that primitive orienting tendencies are innate activity patterns, which we are able to inhibit by a variety of cognitive processes as well as by anchoring ourselves to the environment. There are many anecdotes of what happens when we are deprived of cues. In the desert, people turn right full circle. In approaching mausoleums where there are steps on the left and steps on the right, they choose the right. In the animal literature, there are experiments showing that if you blind certain insects they will not fly straight, but they curve to one side, and this is stable and characteristic of a species (8).

So, exact symmetry is something that only engineers can achieve. Nature cannot be quite that subtle. I propose that in humans the tendency to explore to the right is greater than that to explore to the left. If that is the case, it should be apparent in the least sophisticated humans available for study, namely newborn babies. And it is known that newborn babies orient about four times as frequently to the right as to the left in their spontaneous behavior (12,14).

For a variety of human performance and neurological reasons, we think of the left hemisphere as being more potent in approach programming, although both hemispheres are obviously capable of programming both approach and withdrawal. This could be a rationale for the preponderance of neglect with right-hemisphere lesions. In other words, a right-hemisphere lesion could release a more potent approach tendency to the right side, based on unopposed action by the left hemisphere.

Let us now review briefly the effect of lesions selective for one or the other side, and remind ourselves that if one side of the brain is damaged the other takes over to the extreme of its behavioral range. This is dramatically illustrated in the Wada Test, in which a barbiturate is injected into one carotid artery to determine the side of language dominance (15). One hemisphere is temporarily inactivated. In concert with the drooping of the contralateral arm, there is a swing of the eyes to the side of the injection, the eyes going to the extreme of lateral gaze. Each hemisphere is in control of contralateral gaze. If you inactivate the right hemisphere, the eyes turn right. The left hemisphere causes that by becoming disinhibited with respect to its role within a reciprocal system. So, we propose that there is a reciprocal relation between right and left gaze, which is demonstrable via the cortical control centers in the way I have mentioned. This, however, does not explain how the inhibition is transmitted. Perhaps there is a system in which the hemispheres reciprocally relate through the corpus callosum or a system in which interaction is carried on through brainstem centers. Although we have not yet resolved this issue, I suspect that most, if not all, of this inhibitory traffic is at a brainstem rather than at a callosal level (7). The reason, as Pasik pointed out by implication, is that when you cut the corpus callosum you do not disorganize lateral eye movements *(this volume)*. Lateral gaze is still coordinated to right and left.

In a series of experiments that I carried out with Colwyn Trevarthen, with the aid of an ingenious eye movement apparatus that he devised, we looked at lateral attending in callosally sectioned patients. Let me briefly illustrate the nature of the effect of callosal section on hemispheric relations with a report of two experiments. The first involves a simple visual search paradigm (9). A letter is flashed in one or the other half field, or in both simultaneously. The subject simply responds affirmatively if it is the letter "K" but not if it is some other letter. The positive instance may appear on the right or on the left, or on both sides simultaneously for all the subject knows.

We took latency and error scores, but our latencies were perfectly valueless because of the high incidence of errors. We found that there was a tremendous incidence of total misses of the positive instance, when it came to the left half field. Later I will model this for you with respect to the interaction of orientor and processor within a hemisphere. But, first, I will refer to another of our studies with split-brain patients (13). This was a "completion" experiment in which we showed simple shapes (half a square, half a circle, etc.) and half words (the beginning of a word or the end of a word briefly exposed in one or the other half field). Exposure of incomplete forms or words, so as to overlap the impaired side of the visual field to patients with unilateral parietal lesions, causes completion (16). That completion takes the form of a "whole report." The subject sees a half-circle as a whole circle. When a subject was shown the letters "ing," he read it as "singing." It is the "end of the display" phenomenon that I referred to earlier. An interesting new finding was that one did not have to put the half figure at the midline (11). Even if it was well out in either visual field, the patient would complete it. I bring this up because we also did this with the split-brain subjects and found that they completed across the midline. If you exposed three sides of a square in the right half field, the split-brain subject would report a full square or select one from a recognition ensemble. Stimuli away from the midline in each half field were completed toward the other side. We conclude from this experiment that each hemisphere generates information from a biased information retrieval system, such that information to one side is given more weight than that to the other side. If something is presented to the left of something else, the left hemisphere misses it. If something is missing from the left side of a display, the left hemisphere does not notice that it is missing, which is just the obverse of a neglect logic. Completion is not noticing that something is not there.

The phenomena of lateral attending do not occur only in response to external stimulation. Rather, there is an intimate and lawful relationship between the laterality of the cognitive processor in use, and where one is looking. When normal right-handed subjects were given verbal problems to solve, they would look to the right when thinking of them, whereas they would look to the left while thinking about spatial problems (5) or more up than to the left, reflecting possibly bilateral spreading of a spatial map across the hemispheres, or bilaterally with a superimposed asymmetrical component. But the basic demonstration was that if a person adopts a lateralized mental set, physiologically he has to activate the appropriate hemisphere, which then emits its orientation response, one component of which happens to be right-looking. Stimulation comes in to the visual area of the left brain, for example, from the right half field. This triggers a corticofugal influence that goes to the brainstem and then causes a corticopetal selective activation of the appropriate processor used for processing that category of input. That activation also has effect on the orientor of that side, causing a swing to the right. Now, the interesting aspect of all this is that you can leave out the first step. If something does happen in the right visual field, one can analyze and sufficiently categorize it to decide whether to adopt a verbal or spatial set, and then the brainstem prepares the appropriate mechanism for action. However, we argue that the same set of connections can be used for adopting a more spontaneous mental set. So, if one happens to have adopted a verbal set, his left-hemisphere processor is activated and his eyes turn to the right. Conversely, if one turns on his rightward or leftward orientor, as if to track a stimulus, it appears one also activates other areas of the same hemisphere. This implies that if one turns to the right, he is better able to think in words than if he turns to the left. In a recent experiment (9), we gave subjects a reaction time test that had a crucial spatial ingredient in terms of pattern matching. We had them do it immediately after having them swing head, eyes, and shoulders around 90° either to the left or to the right, and found that they responded with shorter latency when they had swung left. This had been predicted on the basis that swinging left would activate the right hemisphere, which would then be more prepared to deal with what was, in fact, its specialized responsibility, the pattern matching that followed.

Many experiments illustrate that adopting a lateralized mental set has lateralized consequences on the direction of selective attention (3,5,6,9), and a second model is derived to account for the bias in the prevalence of left-sided neglect over right (4). Let us consider how the clinician approaches the affected patient. Clearly, the patient initially adopts a verbal set on hearing what the clinician is saying and responding to what he is saying. This activates the left hemisphere, as if one were applying an electrode to that structure. Now, let us suppose that there is an antecedent imbalance, and then consider the consequences of that behavioral activation on the imbalance, depending on its direction. Say the subject has a right-hemisphere lesion. Already there is an imbalance, so he has an orienting tendency to the right, much more than to the left. We now stimulate the left hemisphere by putting it into verbal activation. This exaggerates the neglect of the left side and gives rise to the gross phenomena. Consider, however, a patient who has his imbalance the other way, owing to a left-sided lesion: he has a left-looking tendency and little ability to orient to the right. If he drifts into a verbal set, this will somewhat strengthen the countervailing tendency, oppose his pathological bias, and mitigate the clinical neglect phenomena. Admittedly, this is hypothesis. I have no experimental data to show that the degree of elicited neglect is a function of the mental set at the time of measurement, but Heilman and colleagues have recently accomplished such a demonstration *(this volume)*.

A final point. Turning to the right not only is approach to the right but also is turning away from the left. In neglect, it is not always clear what is happening. Is the patient turning right or is he turning away from the left? They are not quite the same thing. Now, in the nervous system, there is progressive abstraction; at a low level, very concrete behavior is represented, such as physical approach and withdrawal, and, at successively higher levels, these become increasingly abstracted. For instance, at the highest level of processing, approach could be euphoria and withdrawal could be depression. And, withdrawal could include being contemptuous of one's left arm or leg, or the clinician on one's left. Again, this is purely speculative, but Weinstein cites many observations that can be conceptualized as abstracted withdrawal at a highly elaborated level.

To summarize, I propose that unilateral neglect of space represents an imbalance in lateral orienting tendencies, with excessive orienting toward the side of the lesion and deficient orienting away from the lesion.

REFERENCES

1. Hecaen, H. (1969): Aphasic, apraxic and agnosic syndromes in right and left hemisphere lesions. In: *Handbook of Clinical Neurology,* Vol. 4, edited by P. J. Vinken and G. W. Bruyn. North Holland, Amsterdam.
2. Kinsbourne, M. (1966): Limitations in visual capacity due to cerebral lesions. *Proc. 18th Int. Congr. Psychol.,* pp. 120–127. University Press, Moscow.
3. Kinsbourne, M. (1970): The cerebral basis of lateral asymmetries in attention. *Acta Psychol.,* 33:193–201.
4. Kinsbourne, M. (1970): A model for the mechanism of unilateral neglect of space. *Trans. Am. Neurol. Assoc.,* 95:143–145.
5. Kinsbourne, M. (1972): Eye and head turning indicate cerebral lateralization. *Science,* 176: 539–541.
6. Kinsbourne, M. (1973): The control of attention by interaction between the cerebral hemispheres. In: *Attention and Performance IV,* edited by S. Kornblum. Academic Press, New York.
7. Kinsbourne, M. (1974): Lateral interactions in the brain. In: *Hemispheric Disconnection and Cerebral Function,* edited by M. Kinsbourne and W. L. Smith. Charles C Thomas, Springfield, Ill.
8. Kinsbourne, M. (1974): Mechanisms of hemispheric interaction in man. In: *Hemispheric Disconnection and Cerebral Function,* edited by M. Kinsbourne and W. L. Smith. Charles C Thomas, Springfield, Ill.
9. Kinsbourne, M. (1975): The mechanism of hemispheric control of the lateral gradient of attention. In: *Attention and Performance V,* edited by P. M. A. Rabbitt and S. Dornic. Academic Press, London.
10. Kinsbourne, M. (1977): The biological determinants of functional bisymmetry and asymmetry. In: *The Asymmetrical Function of the Brain,* edited by M. Kinsbourne. Cambridge University Press, New York. *(In press.)*

11. Kinsbourne, M., and Warrington, E. K. (1962): A variety of reading disability associated with right hemisphere lesions. *J. Neurol. Neurosurg. Psychiatry,* 25:339–344.
12. Siqueland, E. R., and Lipsitt, L. P. (1966): Conditioned head turning in human newborns. *J. Exp. Child Psychol.,* 4:356–377.
13. Trevarthen, C. W. (1974): Functional relations of disconnected hemispheres with the brainstem, and with each other: monkey and man. In: *Hemispheric Disconnection and Cerebral Function,* edited by M. Kinsbourne and W. L. Smith. Charles C Thomas, Springfield, Ill.
14. Turkewitz, G., Gordon, B. W., and Birch, M. G. (1968): Head turning in the human neonate: Effect of prandial condition and lateral preference. *J. Comp. Physiol. Psychol.,* 59:189–192.
15. Wada, J., and Rasmussen, T. R. (1960): Intracarotid amytal for the lateralization of cerebral speech dominance. *J. Neurosurg.,* 17:266–282.
16. Warrington, E. K. (1962): The completion of visual forms across hemianopic field defects. *J. Neurol. Neurosurg. Psychiatry,* 25:208–217.

DISCUSSION

Dr. Pasik: Because you have been careful not to mention by name any anatomic structure, such as the brainstem, may I coax you to do so? What do you think of the output from the basal ganglia? We and others have made many unilateral lesions in the brain and have produced circling behavior. But the maximum, most potent, circling behavior results from a lesion that will eliminate the output from the basal ganglia system. The lesion involves the inner pallium or section of the ansa lenticularis. Do you have any ideas on this?

Dr. Kinsbourne: I think you are right. I see the basal ganglia system in relation to the activation of motor behavior, which is in balance in terms of directional turning tendencies. However, the anatomical pathways are outside my area of expertise. I might make one point about specificity. At the behavioral level, virtually any hemispheric lesion will cause an imbalance. For example, take dichotic listening. If you give simultaneous verbal messages with different content, the normal subject, with his left hemisphere specialized for language, does better with right-ear input. However, if you have a lesion in the left hemisphere, then the asymmetry is reversed. In this case, you do better with the left ear than with the right. This effect is not due to damaging specifically the left-hemisphere auditory connections, because it doesn't matter where the left-hemisphere lesion is. It can even be frontal. Therefore, there is a balance of activation between the hemispheres as a whole that influences particular processes wherever they are along it.

Dr. Weinstein: The idea of mutually interacting directional forces with a rightward bias is appealing, and provides a quite plausible explanation for the predominance of left-sided neglect. However, why doesn't the principle operate in cases of extinction? The incidence of visual and tactile extinction yields no left-right difference, that is, we find right-sided extinction just as frequently as we find left-sided extinction.

My second question concerns the degree of the preponderance of left-sided full-fledged hemi-inattention over right-sided neglect. If this is based on a universal dextral turning tendency, then the relative incidence should be on the order of the predominance of right handedness over left handedness. But, in our experience, the considerable number of cases of conspicuous right-sided neglect far exceeds the proportions for left-brain and right-brain dominance.

Also, in relation to the proposition that the patient is adopting a verbal set and activating his left hemisphere, it seems to me that, in examining a patient with a serious brain illness, the emotional impact would be at least as important as the verbal one. Dr. Kinsbourne is certainly familiar with the recent paper in *Science* based on his work, which showed that questions involving spatial thought and emotionally loaded questions produced eye shift to the left, whereas verbal concepts had predominant shift to the right.[1]

[1] Schwartz, G. E., Davidson, R. J., and Maer, F. (1975): Right hemisphere lateralization for emotion in the human brain: Interactions with cognition. *Science,* 190:286–288.

Finally, I wonder if the idea of torques and primitive directional forces would explain all the complex and sophisticated manifestations of hemi-neglect. How does it explain the behavior of the patient who ignores his left side, but represents it in drawings, humor, and other forms of metaphor?

Dr. Kinsbourne: That's a considerable attentional challenge. Obviously, I can't answer all of the questions, but they are, none the less, interesting. With regard to the relative incidence of right- and left-sided lesions, at the basic, very mild level that extinction represents, the factors causing imbalance do not work. When the case is aggravated, as in marked hemi-inattention, they come into play. I think the point of emotional mental set is well taken. As Dr. Weinstein reminded us, Gary Schwartz from Harvard has shown that people don't only look left when they think spatially, but also look left when they are upset or when they are given upsetting material. Now you might argue, by my own logic, that you have a patient with a right-hemisphere lesion, and you ask him to do something, you are obviously a scary person to him. You are obviously a doctor after all, and, indeed, even to a normal person, it's terrifying. So why aren't you activating his right hemisphere? And how am I to answer that? Well, he doesn't have a right hemisphere, it's all dead? But, that's an unsatisfactory answer. I do not know. Again, I think the question is beautifully put, and I think it doesn't either speak for or against the argument but rather suggests an experiment, which, after all, is even better.

Dr. Diamond: I got the impression from your model that most of the imbalance would occur in the preparation for stimulation and not in the response. In studying this phenomenon of imbalance some years ago, we found an effect that we referred to as spatial bias. We were able to demonstrate such bias in cases where no stimuli were used. That is to say, in trials during which no stimuli were presented, we found an imbalance, as you put it.

Also, I should mention that many times when there is apparent neglect of a stimulus on one side, there is, nevertheless, an ultimate response given, as for example when the patient is asked, "Where did I touch you?" The subject will inspect his stimulated hand, and finally deny that he was touched, or offer some other verbal evasion. So, imbalance or bias doesn't seem to me to be as much of an afferent mechanism, as you say.

Dr. Kinsbourne: Let me endorse both points in the following way: Indeed, it is a matter of preparation for response because, as I began by saying, a person with a lateralized lesion or an animal will spontaneously explore in a biased way. In other words, he will initiate the search for stimulation in a biased way, showing visual search task in many ways, so you have to be right. I would agree with that. I wouldn't like to partition input and output processing in this particular context. I'd rather think of it as one system and wait until a final decision is made when we know more about it. The answer to your other point is yes. As you pointed out, it would be foolish to try to account for the whole phenomenology of unilateral neglect at a low level of information processing. Dr. Weinstein made the point very clearly. You gave a further instance. By all means, I like to resort to the notion of the same type of behavior at different levels of abstraction. So, what is at a lower level of abstraction, a physical withdrawal or failure to respond, is the high level of abstraction a contemptuous ignoring of or reluctance to talk about whatever it is. These are different aspects of the same type of functional organization. So, I would indeed like to think of the person whom you describe as somebody who was reluctant to talk of the left half of his body. He didn't want to do it. You could perhaps press him into it. Just like the person who has neglect and seems reluctant to look left. You can beat him into it, if you really lay the law down to him. So, ingredients of this behavior seem to be at a very high level. Now, you are going all the way from two little touches to making a contemptuous remark about your own left arm. It sounds awfully different. Whether different lesions invoked these phenomena to different degrees I don't know, but all I can do is to rest with the point that a withdrawal at one or another level would, for the time being, accommodate all these behaviors, in my view.

Dr. Bodis-Wollner: I just wanted some clarification because I heard a lot of agreement between Dr. Heilman and you.

Dr. Kinsbourne: No conspiracy.

Dr. Bodis-Wollner: No, I wouldn't imply that, but yet now, in your answer, I heard something that makes me think that the understanding should, in fact, be clarified more. We didn't hear about your concept of the mechanism or the model of attention. From your answer to Dr. Diamond, my understanding was that in speaking of hemi-inattention you are ready to regard the problems of hemi-inattention as problems in the "readiness" of the brain for incoming stimuli. To be ready for a certain stimulus is, of course, very important in view of some of the cerebral evoked potentials, or should we look at the emitted potentials or readiness potentials, "Bereitschaft potentiale," CNVs, as our electrical correlate of the lateralized dysfunction in hemi-inattention? The question that I am addressing to you now, is the following: Do you see, in that motoric behavior that was found by Dr. Heilman, a problem in the activity response of the organization to a particular stimulus, or as a problem in the potential readiness to act upon the world?

Dr. Kinsbourne: My answer will not be fully satisfactory because I think that there is evidence for both. In other words, I think that neglect phenomena can be demonstrated in response to passively imposed stimulation, which, more likely, the person who works with monkeys is going to do, because you can't really tell those animals what to do "spontaneously." Whereas, in working with human beings one increasingly has the opportunity of observing and even systematizing differential readiness spontaneously, to entertain certain types of behaviors, as you point out. All I can do is to go back to what you may or may not find as a satisfactory initial account, and say that it is conceivably one in the same system that processes input, leads it down to brainstem for a more diffuse activation of brain area, ready to respond both cognitively and in terms of lateral orienting. We might then say that we might eliminate the first half of it, without input or with imagined input and think in terms of readiness to meet an imagined or hallucinated stimulus or contingency.

Advances in Neurology, Vol. 18, edited by E. A. Weinstein and R. P. Friedland. Raven Press, New York © 1977.

Behavioral Disorders Associated with Hemi-Inattention

Edwin A. Weinstein and Robert P. Friedland

Department of Neurology, Mount Sinai Medical School, New York, New York 10029; and Veterans Administration Hospital, Bronx, New York 10468

This chapter deals with the clinical features of hemi-inattention and their relationship to other alterations in behavior and with the issue of the predominance of neglect of the left over the right side of the body and space.

The material is drawn from approximately 200 cases studied over the past 25 years. Some of these observations, published previously (11,13,15–17), will be cited for illustrative purposes. A number of specific problems will be approached from a quantitative analysis of 63 previously unreported cases.

The following manifestations of hemi-inattention were evaluated:

(a) Visual or tactile extinction brought out by the method of double simultaneous stimulation (DSS). Patients were also tested for cross-modal extinction, usually by an auditory stimulus to one ear and a touch on the opposite hand.

(b) Omission of letters, numbers, or words on one side of a page when patient is asked to read. Omission on one side when patient is asked to tell what is in a picture.

(c) Failure to pick up coins or cards on either the left or right end of a horizontal row.

(d) Omissions, distortions, and asymmetries in drawings of a clock, house, tree, and human figure.

(e) Asymmetry in line bisection.

(f) Failure to respond to auditory stimuli, such as people talking from one side of a room. Failure to notice people on one side.

(g) Failure to raise one arm in response to instructions to raise both arms. Failure to identify body parts only on one side.

(h) Failure to grasp both ear lobes on command (in the absence of marked weakness).

(i) Failure to look in one lateral direction in pursuit or on command in the absence of oculomotor palsy.

(j) Shift of eyes in a lateral direction on exposure to paired visual stimuli, usually the examiner's hands. Patient is not asked to fixate, but simply asked "what do you see?" The shift occurs even when the stimuli are placed in the patient's good visual field.

ALTERATIONS OF BEHAVIOR

Verbal Representations of Neglect

These included explicit and implicit forms of verbal denial such as delusions and confabulations about the affected side of the body and/or that side of space. We also recorded the occurrence of figures of speech (such as metaphor, personification, metonymy, simile, and irony), humor, slang, imagery, and anecdotes to represent one side of the body and/or space. For example, a hemiparetic patient repeatedly expressed the conviction that the city should remit one-half of the taxes on his home because of depreciation. All of these forms of language are grouped under the general heading of metaphor.

Disorientation

All patients were examined for disorientation for place, time, and persons. In disorientation for place, the patient misnames or mislocates the hospital, usually to a site near his home or place of business. The disoriented patient usually maintains his error despite cues, clues, and corrections. Even though the name of the hospital is in full view, the patient rejects the examiner's prompting and persists in his idiosyncratic designation. On occasion, the name given to the hospital is a symbolic representation of a disability, as in the case of a hemiplegic man who called the Bronx Veterans Hospital, located near the Kingsbridge Armory, the "Kingsbridge Armory Hospital" and "Kingsbridge Armless Hospital." A woman persisted in calling the hospital "Misericordia" "because that's how I feel."

In disorientation for time of day, the patient similarly persists in erroneous designations and does not search the physical environment for information through which he could orient himself. Thus, the disoriented patient does not look at his watch or at a wall clock. When he is given a watch by the examiner, he often turns the face or transposes the hands in such a way as to read a time approximating his own misstatement. In fact, we have learned in examining any subject, that if he turns to look at his watch when asked the time, he will prove to be oriented. We considered patients who confused morning and afternoon, or afternoon and evening, or A.M. and P.M., as disoriented for time of day. The patient is apt to give a time which fits into some personal activity, such as giving a morning hour after awakening from a nap. One of our subjects would regularly give three o'clock "because that's when my wife comes."

In disorientation for date, the patient persistently gives the wrong month and/or the wrong year. Disorientation for persons involves the misidentification of *other* persons. (We have actually never seen a patient with organic brain disease, except for global aphasics, who could not give his own name.)

Reduplication

Reduplication for place, time, and persons is closely related to disorientation. In reduplication for place, the patient, when asked how many Mount Sinai or Bronx Veterans Hospitals there are, states that there are two or more. One is generally located at the correct address and the "other" elsewhere. Commonly, the "other" hospital is a "branch" or "annex." There are variations, such as the statement that one part of the building serves as a hospital and another as an "apartment" or "office." In reduplication for time, the patient falsely states that a current event, such as an operation or previous admission, has also occurred previously. Reduplication for time can thus be regarded as an enduring déjà vu phenomenon. Reduplication for persons is the assigning of two identities to the same individual and is usually difficult to separate from temporal reduplication. Thus, the patient states that the nurse on the floor is a girl that he knew back in his home town. Reduplication for parts of the body may also occur, as in the instance of patients who claim to have two left arms or several heads.

It is important to stress that these phenomena are frequently elicited only if the patient is specifically asked the question. A patient may appear to be oriented for place, giving the name and address of the hospital correctly, but when asked if there is another Mount Sinai or Bronx Veterans Hospital in New York, will state there is a hospital so named at some other location.

Aphasia

Testing for aphasic language deficits included evaluation of comprehension, fluency, recitation, repetition, object- and body-part naming, and word patterning. The last involved the ability to give rhymes, alliterations, and homonyms (19).

Topographical Orientation and Dressing Praxis

These were tested in the usual fashion.

Nonaphasic Misnaming

In nonaphasic misnaming (14,18), objects germane to personal experiences and problems are selectively misnamed. These objects include wheelchair, plastic straw, bedrail, hospital bed, doctor's bag, bandage, and surgical glove. Thus, a wheelchair has been called a "swivel chair," a "deck chair," and a "stroller." Such patients are not aphasic. They comprehend well, do not make errors in conversational speech, recite, repeat, and name non-illness-connected objects well. As in the case of disorientation and reduplication, the patient usually persists in his misnaming despite correction.

Proverb Interpretation

We have used the interpretation of idioms and proverbs as an index of the ability to use metaphor. Patients were asked to interpret ten of the following idioms and proverbs: "swell-headed," "tight-fisted," "getting a cold shoulder," "seeing eye to eye," "caught flat-footed," "birds of a feather flock together," "too many cooks spoil the broth," "you can lead a horse to water, but you can't make him drink," "Rome wasn't built in a day," "people in glass houses shouldn't throw stones," and "empty barrels make the most noise." The answers were scored in two ways: as correct or incorrect, and according to whether the response was self-referential (SR) or not. A self-referential answer is the representation of some personal idiosyncratic matter, especially relative to the disability. Thus, following a craniotomy, a patient might interpret "empty barrels make the most noise" as "it means your brains are still rattling around." Such self-referential responses are not to be considered as evidence of "concrete" thinking. They are highly meaningful and no more "concrete" than is humor (10). Secondly, they are highly selective and the patient who interprets "swell-headed" as "your head is all swelled up" translates many other proverbs successfully. The interpretation "your head is all swelled up" would be scored as both incorrect and SR. A response like "patients of the same kind are placed on the same ward" to "birds of a feather. . . ." is rated as correct and SR.

Mood Changes

Evaluation of mood is an artifact of the doctor–patient interaction and is, in part, the expression of how the patient makes the observer feel. Ludic[1] patients make an observer feel euphoric; one is depressed by depressed patients and angered or upset by paranoid ones. Whereas a patient can be regarded as euphoric by some, others feel that there is an underlying depression. Certain observers may consider a patient's joking as part of a euphoria, whereas others consider it sarcasm.

With these reservations, we classed patients' moods as: appropriate; apathetic; ludic and euphoric; paranoid and angry; and withdrawn, depressed, and hypokinetic. We also noted the use of syntax. Ludic patients frequently use the second grammatical person, responding to a doctor's question about their condition with "how is *your* arm, doctor?" Patients with explicit verbal denial often used the third grammatical person: "*the* arm doesn't work," "*they* think it's weak."

OBSERVATIONS

Sixty-three patients were classified according to the side of the unilateral inattention and according to whether the manifestations were mild or minimal, or

---

[1] This is a term used by Jean Piaget to describe the play and imitative aspects of the behavior of young children. It is an apt way to indicate the comic and tragic, or comicotragic, melodramatic behavior present in many patients.

severe or conspicuous. Under the heading of mild or minimal hemi-inattention are included patients with only tactile and visual extinction, and with eye shift on DSS. The group labeled as severe included, in addition, the more conspicuous signs, such as asymmetries in line bisection and drawing, lateralized omissions in reading and looking at pictures, end of display omissions in picking up coins and cards, failure to look to one side on command and in pursuit, failure to grasp both ears, and other gross clinical signs of neglect. While all subjects in both the mild and severe groups showed unimodal extinction, cross-modal extinction (28 cases) occurred only in the severe group. No patient had all the signs of conspicuous neglect. We classed as "severe" those patients who had at least one of the above in consistent fashion for at least a week.

Table 1 shows that there was no significant right-left difference in the cases of mild or minimal hemi-inattention (extinction and eye shift) but a preponderance of left-sided neglect in the cases of conspicuous hemi-inattention.

In Tables 2 and 3, the relationships of the associated disturbances of behavior in left- and right-sided hemi-inattention, respectively, are recorded. The outstand-

TABLE 1. *Incidence of left and right hemi-inattention by severity*

	Right	Left
Mild or minimal	16	15
Severe	12	30

TABLE 2. *Changes in behavior with hemi-inattention*

LEFT HEMI-INATTENTION

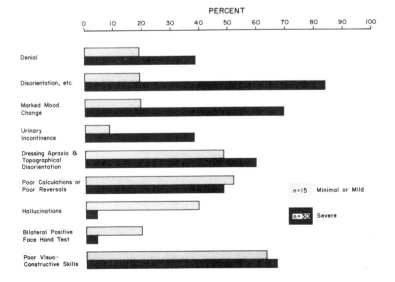

TABLE 3. *Changes in behavior with hemi-inattention*

RIGHT HEMI-INATTENTION

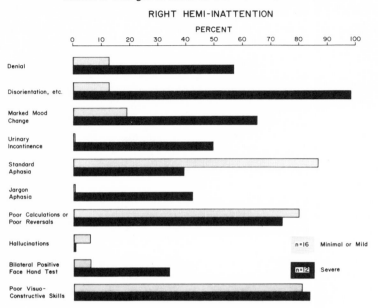

ing finding was that disturbances of consciousness, such as denial, confabulation, reduplicative delusions, nonaphasic misnaming, marked mood changes, and incontinence of urine, occurred significantly more frequently in the severely hemi-inattentive groups, left and right. In other words, while visual and tactile extinction may occur in the absence of disorders of mood and consciousness, severe hemi-neglect is almost always associated with disturbances in mood and consciousness.[2]

In contrast, the incidence of visuoconstructional defects (apart from neglect), topographical disorientation, and dressing apraxia was no greater in cases of severe hemi-inattention than in those with minimal neglect. This suggests that, although disorders of consciousness are significantly related to hemi-inattention, visual-constructive disorders are not.

The difference between minimal and pronounced hemi-inattention cannot be explained on the severity of brain damage per se. A bilaterally positive face-hand test, impaired calculations, and spelling reversals are common manifestations of diffuse cortical or cerebral involvement. Such patients could not reverse the

---

[2] Confabulation, reduplication, delusional denial, nonaphasic misnaming, and disorientation are called disturbances of consciousness because they are changes in the interaction of the self in the environment. Personal experiences are represented in terms of events, persons, places, objects, and times, to a degree beyond the awareness of the speaker. In recovery from a prolonged unconsciousness, as after a head injury, a period of disorientation occurs before full consciousness is reached.

spelling of their first names and words like "world." They were unable to calculate the number of nickels in $3 or to do simple sums and subtractions, such as $19 + 94$ and $94 - 19$. Only 1 of the 30 patients with severe left-sided neglect had a bilaterally positive face-hand test, whereas 3 of the 15 minimally hemi-inattentive patients had a positive test.

A special feature of right-sided neglect was aphasia. According to our criteria for aphasic language deficit, 24 of the 28 cases of mild and severe hemi-neglect were aphasic. Among the 14 cases with evidence of aphasia in the minimally hemi-inattentive group, all were standard aphasics. Of the 12 patients with severe hemi-neglect, 5 exhibited jargon. None of the jargon patients had a defect in comprehension so severe that they could not understand questions relating to illness or orientation, or carry out tests of neglect. Thus, some of the same factors that differentiate standard aphasia from jargon are also important in the differentiation of extinction from the more conspicuous types of hemi-inattention.

Table 4 shows the results of idiom and proverb interpretations, calculated to the nearest percent. In the table, right-sided and left-sided inattention are combined so that only two groups are compared, the minimal and the severe. We found that the severely hemi-inattentive group actually obtained better scores in terms of correct–incorrect. This reflects the larger number of aphasic patients in the mild right-sided hemi-inattention group. The more striking finding is the tremendous difference in the incidence of SR responses that occurred almost exclusively in patients with conspicuous hemi-neglect, right and left. In summary, mild right hemi-inattention tends to have low correct and low SR scores, severe right hemi-neglect has low correctness and high SR, mild left hemi-inattention has high correctness and low SR, and conspicuous left hemi-inattention has high correctness and high SR.

Thus, for conspicuous right-sided hemi-inattention to exist, the patient must have a disturbance in mood and/or consciousness and, like the subject with severe left-sided neglect, must be either nonaphasic or have either jargon aphasia or one of its analogues, such as verbal stereotypy, marked perseveration, "officialese," or marked withdrawal (20,21).

An interesting feature of this study was the paucity of hallucinations in the conspicuously hemi-inattentive group. This might be explained with the supposition that episodic disturbances of consciousness do not occur when there is a continuous impairment of consciousness. Thus, hallucinations in the left field, for example, bear the same relationship to more enduring unilateral neglect that

TABLE 4. *Proverb interpretation*

	Severe hemi-inattention (left and right combined)	Minimal hemi-inattention (left and right combined)
% Correct responses	78	58
% SR responses	31	1

TABLE 5. *Extinction vs hemi-neglect*

Extinction	Hemi-neglect
Nonsymbolic	Symbolic
Nonselective	Selective
Unimodal	Cross-modal
No lateralized predominance	Lateralized predominance
Enduring	More transient
No associated disorders of consciousness necessary	Associated disorders of consciousness
Seizures, hallucinations may occur	Seizures and hallucinations rare
Standard aphasia, if aphasic	Jargon aphasia frequent, if aphasic

déjà vu episodes bear to temporal reduplication. This hypothesis is strengthened by the observation that seizures, likewise, are uncommon in severe hemi-neglect.

Table 5 summarizes the differences between extinction and what we have called severe neglect.

DISCUSSION

There appear to be at least two mechanisms in hemi-inattention. The first is that of extinction and eye shift and the second is the process of symbolization involved in gesture and metaphor. Extinction and eye shift may be regarded as forms of sensory and motor interaction in which simultaneous activation of the hemispheres impairs the function of the lesioned hemisphere so that a lateralized sensory or motor deficit appears. Eye shift is the motor analog of sensory extinction.

This formulation, however, does not explain the predominance of right-hemisphere lesions and the consistent association of disturbances of consciousness and metaphorical speech with conspicuous hemi-inattention. In our view, the ratio of left- to right-sided hemi-inattention will vary with the richness and complexity of the symbolism in which the manifestations are expressed. Extinction and eye shift have very little meaning in terms of the expression of feelings and emotions. The manifestations of conspicuous hemi-neglect, on the other hand, involving metaphor and gesture, are highly symbolic in an experiential sense. It follows that if extinction and eye shift are the sole criteria of hemi-neglect, there should be no difference between left and right, which is precisely what was found. It is the experience of most neurologists that visual and tactile extinction occur as frequently on the right side of the body as on the left. In auditory extinction, there is similarly no predominance of left-sided hemi-inattention with hemispheric lesions (1,7). Similarly, hemi-inattention, produced experimentally in animals by a great variety of lesions, has shown no predilection for either side.

The predominance of left-sided over right-sided hemi-neglect in the literature ranges from 3 to 1 to 16 to 1 in case series. It is evident that the incidence depends on what criteria for hemi-inattention are used. If one goes through individual case reports, it is unusual to find a case of right-sided neglect. The reason seems to be that individual cases are more apt to be accepted for publication if they have some unique or spectacular feature, such as that of a man who moved the pieces only on one side of the chess board. Another reason for the great predominance of left-sided hemi-inattention is that patients with left-hemisphere lesions and right hemiparesis tend to be eliminated from consideration if asymmetry of figure drawing is the main criterion. Similarly, subjects with left-hemisphere lesions may have such severe visuoconstructive defects and poor drawings that it is difficult to detect asymmetry. Finally, there is the question of examiner bias. One may be so convinced by textbook statements that hemi-inattention is a pathognomonic sign of a right-parietal lesion that he may not search as assiduously for signs of right-sided neglect.

This study shows that disturbances of consciousness are usually related to conspicuous hemi-neglect, but topographical disorientation and dressing apraxia, although common in parietal lobe lesions, are not. This indicates that involvement of the limbic reticular system is necessary for the enduring existence of marked hemi-inattention, a conclusion borne out by the character of the lesions (see Introduction, and Chapter 7). We have used the terms disturbances of consciousness and disturbances of metaphorical speech more or less interchangeably, because in each there is a change in the interaction of the self in the environment and in the way experience is perceived in the symbolic context of the physical world. In confabulation, the patient's feelings and other personal experience are expressed in terms of (fictitious) events, in disorientation they are expressed in terms of date and place, in reduplication in terms of persons, and in nonaphasic misnaming in terms of objects. The analogies to metonymy, personification, and other tropes are obvious.

Turning to the relationship of jargon aphasia to neglect, it has been reported as occurring in association (20); jargon may be regarded as a combination of fluent aphasia and a disturbance of consciousness (12,13). Critchley (4) referred to jargon as anosognosic aphasia. However, while the patient with jargon appears unaware of his speech disturbance and may deny it when specifically asked, some of his language involves an attempt to explain, rationalize, or otherwise symbolically represent his problem. Jargon is, to some degree, selective, and, in interviews, the longest answers are elicited in response to questions about illness. Interpretations of proverbs by jargon patients, as we have seen, are highly self-referential. The jargon patient is usually ludic and euphoric and/or paranoid. Patients with standard aphasia, on the other hand, are quite aware of their deficits and do not attempt the low frequency and "high-sounding" words and ornate phraseology in which the jargon patient seeks to give the picture of competent, even eloquent, speech. Thus the behavior of the patient with jargon aphasia shows many resemblances to that of the person with a right-hemisphere lesion with hemi-inattention, denial, confabulation, disorientation, and mood changes. This observation should give pause to those writers who, on the gross evidence of hemispheric lesions, claim that the left hemisphere subserves language and the right, emotion.

A striking feature of conspicuous hemi-inattention, left and right, is that the patient persists in neglecting one side and even denies its ownership, but at the same time he represents it in metaphorical speech and in gesture. He is aware of the side in one context and not another. For example, one of our patients with a left hemiplegia neglected his left arm and denied it was paralyzed but called it "a canary claw, yellow and shrivelled." Thus, he did not recognize his left side in a referential context but he did in the experiential symbolic mode of an emotionally laden metaphor.[3]

This selectivity has its analog in some important experiments by Mountcastle (8) in monkeys. Mountcastle found special cells in the parietal association areas, 5 and 7, of the monkey which fired only when certain motivated actions were carried out on the contralateral side. Area 5 cells fired only if the movement of the contralateral arm satisfied some appetitive drive, such as securing food, grooming, or touching a switch that brought a liquid reward. Other visual, auditory, or somatic sensory stimuli did not activate the cells. Certain Area 7 cells were fired when the monkey fixed his gaze on food when he was hungry or looked at a target that brought liquid refreshment when he was thirsty. This work provides significant verification of the important role of motivational factors in hemi-neglect.

Lastly, the findings are relevant to the whole question of the language functions of the brain. Although the so-called language areas are traditionally restricted to a portion of the cortex of the dominant hemisphere with some recent implication of the thalamus, it should be recognized that the limbic reticular system is of comparable importance. The functions of language go beyond comprehension and expression, sound and word categorization, recitation and repetition. Language creates a sense of reality and identity; it not only evokes but shapes our feelings. It does not simply label what we see, feel, and hear, but, to a considerable degree, quite out of our awareness, predetermines our perception of our environment. Metaphor, drama, art, and poetry all transform reality. The right hemisphere is not a linguistically primitive shadow of the left, capable of comprehen-

---

[3] Symbols may be classified as belonging to one of two types, referential or experiential. Referential or universal symbols are meaningful by reason of the relationship of the symbol to the physical referent. Mathematical notations, the Morse Code, and flag signaling devices are examples. Experiential symbols, on the other hand, express feelings, and meaning depends more on context. In a referential sense, the American flag denotes national sovereignty. Experientially, it may express feelings of pride and patriotism in one context, and of hatred and disgust in another. Experiential symbols may be highly condensed. The Scarlet Letter "A," denoted the first letter of the alphabet; connoted shame, sin, and disgrace; and embodied the values of a whole culture. The symbol, in the experiential mode, not only evokes and expresses feelings, but shapes them and reinforces the sense of identity of the users. We are quite conscious of the referential aspects of symbolism but less aware of the processes of interaction in the social environment that determine meaning in the experiential mode.

sion, some naming, and the uttering of four-letter words; by reason of its corticolimbic connections, it is especially involved in the relationships between language and perceptual and emotional processes on which metaphorical speech so largely depends. The question arises as to whether there are anatomical or physiological differences in the corticolimbic connections of the hemispheres. So many metaphors are multimodal that the more diffuse organization of sensory functions in the right hemisphere, reported by Semmes et al. (9), may be relevant to the way metaphor enables us to perceive reality more vividly. This does not mean that we can "localize" metaphor in the minor hemisphere. The superior ability of the dominant hemisphere in maintaining simultaneously different frames of linguistic reference, indicates its important role in the use of metaphor and, of course, humor. Rather than stating that the left hemisphere is dominant for language, it may be more exact to say that the left hemisphere is dominant for the phonological, sequential, syntactic, and referential functions of language, whereas the right hemisphere is more specialized for the experiential aspects of language.

REFERENCES

1. Bender, M. G., and Diamond, S. P. (1965): An analysis of auditory perceptual defects with observations on the localization of dysfunction. *Brain,* 88:675–686.
2. Cohn, R. (1961): *The Person Symbol in Clinical Medicine.* Charles C Thomas, Springfield, Ill.
3. Cohn, R. (1972): Eyeball movements in homonymous hemianopia following simultaneous bitemporal object presentation. *Neurology,* 22:12–14.
4. Critchley, M. (1965): The neurology of psychotic speech. *Br. J. Psychiatry,* 110:353–364.
5. Critchley, M. (1974): Misoplegia or hatred of hemiplegia. *Mt. Sinai J. Med. N.Y.,* 41:1,82–87.
6. Friedland, R. P., and Weinstein, E. A. (1977): Elicitation of hemi-inattention following barbiturate administration. *(In preparation.)*
7. Goodglass, H. (1967): Binaural digit presentation and early lateral brain damage. *Cortex,* III: 295–306.
8. Mountcastle, V. B. (1975): *The World Around Us: Neural Command Functions for Selective Attention.* The F. O. Schmitt Lecture in Neuroscience. Neurosciences research program, bull. 15.
9. Semmes, J., Weinstein, S., Ghent, L., and Teuber, H. L. (1960): *Somatosensory Changes After Penetrating Brain Wounds in Man.* Harvard University Press, Cambridge.
10. Weinstein, E. A. (1974): The neurology of humor. *Mt. Sinai J. Med. N.Y.,* 41:1,235–239.
11. Weinstein, E. A., and Cole, M. (1964): Concepts of anosognosia. In: *Dynamic Neurology,* edited by L. E. Halpern. Jerusalem Post Press, Jerusalem.
12. Weinstein, E. A., Cole, M., Lyerly, O. G., and Ozer, M. N. (1966): Meaning in jargon aphasia. *Cortex,* II:165–187.
13. Weinstein, E. A., Cole, M., Mitchell, M., and Lyerly, O. G. (1964): Anosognosia and aphasia. *Arch. Neurol.,* 10:376–386.
14. Weinstein, E. A., and Kahn, R. L. (1952): Non-aphasic misnaming (paraphasia) in organic brain disease. *Arch. Neurol. Psychiatry,* 67:72–79.
15. Weinstein, E. A., and Kahn, R. L. (1955): *Denial of Illness: Symbolic and Physiological Aspects.* Charles C Thomas, Springfield, Ill.
16. Weinstein, E. A., Kahn, R. L., and Malitz, S. (1956): Confabulation as a social process. *Psychiatry,* 19:383–396.
17. Weinstein, E. A., Kahn, R. L., and Slote, W. (1955): Withdrawal, inattention and pain asymbolia. *Arch. Neurol. Psychiatry,* 74:235–248.
18. Weinstein, E. A., and Keller, N. J. A. (1963): Linguistic patterns of misnaming in brain injury. *J. Neuropsychologia,* 1:79–90.

19. Weinstein, E. A., and Lyerly, O. G. (1974): Word patterning deficits in aphasia. Paper presented at meeting of the Academy of Aphasia, Washington, D.C., October 14, 1974.
20. Weinstein, E. A., and Lyerly, O. G. (1976): Personality factors in jargon aphasia. *Cortex,* XII:122–133.
21. Weinstein, E. A., and Puig-Antich, J. (1974): Jargon and its analogs. *Cortex,* X: (1), 235–239.

Advances in Neurology, Vol. 18, edited by E. A. Weinstein and R. P. Friedland. Raven Press, New York © 1977.

Hemi-Inattention in Rehabilitation: The Evolution of a Rational Remediation Program

Leonard Diller and Joseph Weinberg

Institute of Rehabilitation Medicine, New York University Medical Center, New York, New York 10016

This chapter describes a research program that was designed to elucidate problems of hemi-inattention as seen in the context of a medical rehabilitation setting. Out of this program, an approach to the amelioration of many of the problems found in patients with hemi-inattention was developed. Before proceeding, we will briefly comment on the current status of the field from a rehabilitation perspective.

Medical rehabilitation aims to prepare the patient for independence by training in functional activities of daily living. Diagnosis and symptom description are directed not merely to the disease process but also to overcoming the disabilities consequent to the disease. If the patient exhibits cognitive deficits on psychometric test performance, produces bizarre reproductions of drawings, and/or appears too restless to be tested, how can independence be increased? On the one hand, most efforts in rehabilitation are directed at treating motor deficits. On the other hand, most of the work in neuropsychology stops at the point of diagnosis and symptom description without attending to issues of remediation and rehabilitation. This creates a vacuum in theory and technique and fails to address the question. On reflection, it can be seen that this vacuum carries over in dealing with phenomena of hemi-inattention or spatial neglect in rehabilitation. Few systematic attempts have been made to examine hemi-inattention as a problem encountered while retraining individuals undergoing rehabilitation.

There is an absence of data on the natural history of hemi-inattention. Most descriptions of hemi-inattention are accounts of patients on neurology services who are seen shortly after the onset of brain damage when they may still be mentally confused. Anosognosia, for example, a phenomenon which appears along with mental confusion, is rare in rehabilitation programs. Manifestations of hemi-inattention in rehabilitation may be seen in the following examples: (a) Disturbances in grooming whereby men omit parts of the face while shaving, women misapply makeup, and both mismatch clothing. (b) Difficulty in telling time from a clock and/or disorientation for time because of an inability to read a program schedule card. (c) Difficulty in dialing a telephone or making sense of a TV show or movie, and problems in reading, copying, and arithmetic. (d)

Frequency of accidents while on rehabilitation programs (5). (e) Difficulty in shopping, making change, and returning to work (14). (f) Medical complications. We know of a diabetic, left hemiplegic individual who consistently omitted checking off the left side of his daily menu resulting in a dietary deficiency that led to grand mal seizure. (g) Problems in behaviors such as ambulation and dressing (6,9) that form core criteria for admission and discharge in rehabilitation. (h) On a more subtle level, hemi-inattention may indirectly influence rehabilitation goals leading to premature discharge from rehabilitation programs.

Although some experimental evidence suggests that certain phenomena associated with hemi-inattention, e.g., double simultaneous stimulation (DSS), are amenable to change under coaching (15), there are no data regarding generalization or the practical value of such training. The intensive case studies of Lawson (8) and Luria (10) suggest that improvement might be achieved but that, once the patient's condition has stabilized, interventions are laborious (requiring years of effort). Furthermore, there is a lack of a clear relationship to more general principles of remediation. Therapeutic application of such training techniques would, therefore, appear to yield a meager payoff for a great deal of effort. This discouraging impression has been supported by one of the few controlled studies of perceptual retraining in brain-damaged adults undergoing rehabilitation (11). The results of that study indicated that individuals with right-brain damage and left hemiplegia or hemiparesis resulting from cerebrovascular accident (CVA) who were administered an intensive remediation program did not improve more than a control group on a battery of perceptual tasks.

Our approach to the problem went through four stages:

1. Development of a standard task sensitive to the presence of hemi-inattention.
2. Examination of response styles to determine factors which help elucidate many of the seemingly inexplicable and bizarre features apparent to the observer.
3. Development of a method of determining those task conditions that facilitate or obscure the presence of hemi-inattention.
4. Development of a method (a) to make patients aware of their deficit and (b) to assist them in overcoming the deficit while performing a skilled activity.

In order to accomplish these goals, we have implemented an active research program in our setting that has been translated into a program for the diagnosis and remediation of hemi-inattention. These efforts have been directed primarily at individuals with right-brain damage (RBD) due to CVA.

THE DEVELOPMENT OF A METHOD FOR ASSESSING HEMI-INATTENTION

Visual cancellation tasks were devised that contained letters (N = 600) typed on six lines. The letter "H" served as a target for the subject to cancel. The targets

(N = 105) were so arranged that there were an equal number on different segments of the page (so that one could compare performance on the left side of the page with that on the right); they differed in proximity to each other; and the instructions could be varied to increase the information load by having subjects cancel more than a single letter.

Using this tool in a series of studies with hemiplegic patients in our rehabilitation setting resulted in the following information:

(a) Although some left-brain-damaged (LBD) individuals exhibited hemi-inattention, the occurrence was far less frequent than in RBDs. We cannot extrapolate generalizations about issues of laterality from our data, however, since there may be selective biases in patient selection for rehabilitation; and a number of LBDs have problems of severe aphasia that may have interfered with performance. We, therefore, concentrated our efforts on RBDs.

(b) Forty percent of RBDs have marked hemi-inattention (as observed on the cancellation tasks). Approximately 40% do not exhibit a disturbance and the remainder show traces of a disturbance.

(c) Hemi-inattention is correlated with the presence of a visual field defect but is not synonymous with it, i.e., some individuals exhibit one without the other.

(d) The particular target stimuli, e.g., letters, were not a factor in performance, since similar results were obtained for numbers, shapes, words, and pictures.

RESPONSE CHARACTERISTICS AND TEST CORRELATES ASSOCIATED WITH HEMI-INATTENTION PERFORMANCE ON VISUAL CANCELLATION TASKS

RBDs exhibited several response characteristics:

1. Errors were always those of omission, never of commission.
2. Errors appeared more frequently on the side of the page contralateral to the brain damage than on the ipsilateral side.
3. Many bizarre responses occurred. Some patients began canceling targets in the middle of the page, some skipped around the page, some went in a vertical rather than horizontal direction, some began at the left and went across the page at the top line in a left to right direction, but on the next line moved in a right to left direction.
4. Many patients appeared to perform the task quickly but inaccurately. This finding was of particular interest since LBDs for the most part tended to perform accurately but very slowly.

PERFORMANCE ON OTHER TASKS

The findings of the series of studies also indicated that there appear to be two or possibly three subgroups of RBDs who might be characterized in terms of the presence and extent of hemi-inattention in severe form, in mild form, or not readily observable. The criterion for hemi-inattention was performance on the cancellation task. The subgroups performed differently on a wide variety of tasks, including the following:

1. Wide Range Reading Test
2. Wide Range Arithmetic Test
3. Paragraph Reading (Gray Oral Reading Test)
4. Copying an address
5. Counting faces in a graduation picture
6. Matching faces (3)
7. Digit Span Backwards (12)
8. Object Assembly (WAIS)
9. Picture Completion (WAIS)
10. Face-Hand Test (1)
11. Visual Confrontation (Denny-Brown)
12. Motor Impersistence-Visual (7)
13. Bender-Gestalt
14. Bisecting lines (with differing conditions, loci, and sizes)
15. Locating the center of one's own body (when touched on the back)

Tasks 1, 2, 3, 6, 8, 9, 11, and 13 were taken from standard tests with visual task demands, whereas tasks 4, 5, and 14 were devised specifically for our study. Most of the tasks were visual, but tasks 7, 10, 12, and 15 were not. The nonvisual tasks were included because they were thought to be sensitive to some of the response styles noted above, e.g., a distinct preference was noted for stimuli presented to the right side of space. In observing patients on cancellation tasks, not only were they correct more often on the right side of space, but they acted almost as if the hand holding the pencil was being pulled to the right. We, therefore, devised tool 15 as a measure of shift in awareness of space on the body. When touched on the back, the patient tended to displace the location of his backbone to the right.

It is important to note that in one of the studies the groups did *not* differ on a number of tasks that we postulated were not sensitive to phenomena of hemi-inattention. These tasks included the Purdue Pegboard, Vocabulary, Digit Span Forward, and those aspects of Motor Impersistence which do not have a visual component. The Purdue Pegboard, for example, is based on a visual demand which is in the sagittal plane as opposed to the horizontal plane and, therefore, poses few problems in terms of hemi-inattention. If the board is turned at a 90° angle so that the patient is confronted with the same task on the plane parallel to the horizontal plane, he does poorly. We, therefore, cannot attribute the difficulty to a general cognitive or even perceptual impairment. The problem occurs in the prehension of space. Spatial prehension may be necessary in non-visual situations, as we have suggested elsewhere (12).

TASK CONDITIONS SENSITIVE TO HEMI-INATTENTION

Several features of the cancellation task were found to influence the tendency to omit stimuli.

(a) *Locus of the stimuli:* A stimulus on the left side is more likely to be omitted than one on the right.

(b) *Anchoring:* When patients are given either verbal or visual cues to begin each line at the extreme left side of the page before proceeding, improvement is noted. RBDs are more influenced by anchoring from the left side of space than from the right side of space. Both types of anchoring are superior to free style performance.

(c) *Pacing:* Once the patient is anchored, there is still a tendency to rapid drifting toward targets on the right side of the page. The patient can slow down his performance to an even pace simply by reciting the targets out loud. This automatically harnesses the speed of performance.

(d) *Density:* Errors tended to occur when targets were closer to each other. It is possible to reduce errors by increasing distance between targets. This phenomenon has also been noted by Bender and Diamond (2).

TREATMENT

As in any problem-solving activity, the first step in the treatment of hemi-inattention is to make the patient aware of the problem. This is particularly difficult in hemi-inattention since this failure in awareness appears to be at the heart of the patient's difficulty. If one asks a patient with spatial neglect to turn his head to view a stimulus, he may perform correctly and even report on the stimulus. If one repeats the task, the patient fails and seems oblivious to his previous correct performance. The previous instructions that led to successful performance were not incorporated in his awareness and, therefore, do not carry over. In clinical management, it is important to have the patient recognize his failure in order to get him to deal with the problem. For example, in learning to transfer from a wheelchair a patient must lock his wheelchair on the left side. The patient must first be aware of the brake on the left side. Patients with hemi-inattention typically resist awareness of problems. Such patients may appear negativistic and stubborn.

A number of simple tasks were devised that are designed to foster awareness while at the same time permitting success on simple cueing. Two such tasks are described. In one task a variety of coins and dollar bills is spread in a semicircle on a table before the patient. The patient is asked to pick up the money and hand it to the experimenter. The patient with neglect tends to omit the money in the impaired half of space. The patient is then asked to turn his head to the left to see the money he neglected. He accepts being taught to turn his head to search in this way. In a second task, the patient is asked to copy a simple paragraph or an address. Usually the patient will leave out part of the paragraph or the address. The patient is shown that by turning his head he can see the stimuli he had previously neglected and compensate for his problem.

During this phase of the program, the patient's resistance and suspicions are at a maximum. The examiner must proceed in a cautious yet firm manner. Although we have no data on the question of whether patients with hemi-inattention are in fact aware of the stimuli that they deny exist, the introspections of a number of highly intelligent patients indicate that the individual is aware that something is wrong. He cannot identify the problem and indeed may feel that he is losing his sanity. When this happens he tries doubly hard to cover up the defect in order not to expose himself to others.

OVERCOMING HEMI-INATTENTION

On the basis of the studies in which task conditions sensitive to hemi-inattention were clarified, we postulated that it was possible to train patients to compensate for the difficulties by: (a) Presenting the patient with a task that is sufficiently compelling to cause head turning to the neglected side. (b) Guiding the patient's scanning in a directed, even-paced search of the environment to overcome the "pull" to the right side. (c) Supplying the patient with cues to assist in systematic and orderly scanning and, as the patient improves, gradually reducing cues, so that the patient can perform the activity on his own. (d) Providing feedback to the patient as to the correctness of his performance.

To accomplish the above, an apparatus called "the scanning machine" was devised. This apparatus has two major features. First, it has a target that traverses the perimeter of the board (which is 78" long and 8" wide) at various rates of speed controlled by the trainer. Second, the board is studded with 2 rows of 10 colored lights. The activation of each light is also controlled by a separate button on a panel monitored by the trainer; then lights can be activated singly, in pairs, or in any desired sequence. There are two parts to the use of the machine in training:

1. The patient sits facing the apparatus and is told to look at the target and point to it as it travels around the edge of the board. At the beginning of training, RBD patients with problems in spatial inattention have difficulty finding the target as it traverses the left half of space. The patient's head movement is also slow and jerky as he follows the target. With practice the patient not only turns his head with greater ease and rapidity, but his eyes can follow the target smoothly at varying speeds, regardless of whether the target moves in a right to left or left to right direction. In the beginning of training, it is usually easier for the patient to follow the target from right to left than left to right. When some patients are asked to look at and point to the target that is moving in a right to left direction, the hand will continue across the body midline, while the head and the eyes will stop at the midline. It appears that on his own, the patient has difficulty turning his head and eyes to the impaired side. Thus, in training the

patient to compensate for his inattention to stimuli, one must constantly watch that the patient moves his head to the impaired side. It was also observed that some patients will shift the body or tilt the head to the impaired side while tracking the target. This tendency is discouraged.

2. Another feature of this apparatus is that it contains two rows of colored lights. The lights are used to augment the training by having the patient turn his head and call out the numbers of lights that are on. The training on the light board is usually done in the following sequence: (a) searching for lights in the center; (b) searching for lights on the impaired side; and (c) searching for two or more lights simultaneously on both the impaired and unimpaired side. In training, the patient is told to look for the light/lights on the side that he neglects before searching for the lights on the intact side.

In conjunction with the training on the scanning apparatus, a number of tasks were devised that are used as exercises. One such task is a visual cancellation of numbers in which the patient is asked to cancel out a specific number. The patient is provided with cues, such as a number at the beginning and the end of lines, or a heavy red vertical line is drawn on the side of the page on which the patient shows neglect. This serves as an anchor. The patient is instructed to move his head until the red line is seen and then to continue canceling out the specific stimuli across the lines. The red line is the patient's cue to turn the head to the left and search for the beginning of the line.

The patient's tendency to perform a task quickly, as mentioned before, interferes with the ability to compensate for difficulties and task mastery. Telling the patient to slow down has no effect. While performing on the cancellation tasks, the patient appears to be pulling the hand away from the impaired side and toward the good side. This behavior is controlled by having the patient call out the numbers while canceling them.

An additional visual task involves reading paragraphs from newspapers. The paragraphs are placed on transparencies and projected on the wall so that the stimuli are widely spaced. This makes it easy to notice the stimuli on the impaired side. Large-print editions of *The New York Times* can also be used for exercise in scanning. The training is generally conducted for one session a day for 1 month. We encourage its continuation at home by the patient and the family by using a variety of exercises.

RESULTS

With training periods of 1 hour each day for a 1-month period, the treated groups improved more than controls receiving only traditional occupational therapy for eye-hand skills (4,13). It is possible to train patients with hemi-inattention to improve their performance on reading, copying, and written arithmetic; to improve their performance on tasks of spatial localization and spatial relations; and to improve interpersonal gaze.

Two case studies are presented.

CASE STUDIES

Mr. Z

Mr. Z is a seventy-four year old right-handed male with left hemiparesis secondary to CVA. Up to the time of his stroke, Mr. Z was an active working man with many interests and hobbies. The patient was admitted to the Institute of Rehabilitation Medicine 6 weeks after the onset of the CVA. The findings revealed weakness in muscle power on the left upper and lower extremities, inconsistent responses to sensory stimuli on the left, and inability to ambulate. There was a left homonymous hemianopsia. Visual-motor impersistence was severely deviant. The patient was alert and oriented.

Mr. Z was placed on an active rehabilitation program. He improved in physical therapy,

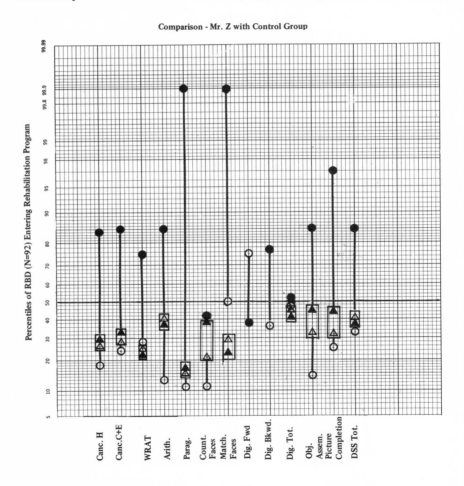

FIG. 1. Comparison of Mr. Z's performance with control group on pre- and post-testing. ○, pre Mr. Z; ●, post Mr. Z; △ pre RBD severe control mean N = 13; ▲ post RBD severe control mean N = 13.

occupational therapy, and activities of daily living. As he was improving, Mr. Z's perceptual problems became of increasing concern. Awareness of neglect of stimuli on the left side, and the problems thus created, made him extremely depressed. Mr. Z found himself no longer able to pursue his favorite pasttimes, reading and following horse-racing results. He felt deprived, useless, and dependent on others. He had difficulty in distinguishing the location of the arms on the face of the watch. Mr. Z needed help with feeding as he constantly neglected food on the left side of his tray. He found TV and movies confusing and unenjoyable. When spoken to, Mr. Z rarely made eye contact. Psychological examination was conducted 10 weeks after the CVA.

Performance on pre- and posttesting for scoreable tests can be seen in Fig. 1. Mr. Z's scores are compared with (a) a subsample of 92 RBDs with left hemiplegia seen in a rehabilitation center, (b) a subsample of 13 RBDs with hemi-inattention who were seen before and after a typical rehabilitation program, where they received the standard treatment used in occupational therapy in our setting. This group has been used as a control group.

The tests include cancellation of letters (single "H" and double "C and E" target), Academic Skills (Wide Range Achievement Test-Reading, Written Arithmetic, Gray Oral Reading Test, and Copying an Address), counting faces in a graduation picture, Matching Faces (3), WAIS Subtests (Digit Span, Object Assembly, Picture Completion), and the Face-Hand Test (DSS). To give the flavor of the performance, we present some of his responses to the tests:

Reading Vocabulary: Wide Range Achievement Test-Reading (WRAT) consists of 10 lines of 75 words of increasing difficulty. Mr. Z severely neglected words on the left side of the page and misread easy words.

Wide Range Achievement Test-Arithmetic: Eight problems of simple subtraction, addition, and multiplication were shown to Mr. Z. He completely omitted the four problems on the left side of the page, and incorrectly calculated the remaining four. Mr. Z added the rows and columns in a disorganized way, ignoring arithmetical signs (Fig. 2). He also omitted numbers.

Reading Comprehension: Seventh grade simple paragraph on the Gray Oral Reading Test. Mr. Z lost his place and became confused. He had difficulty in finding the next line, and he tended to neglect words, particularly on the left side. He could not comprehend what he read, and complained that "nothing seems to make sense anymore" (Fig. 3).

Copying an Address: Mr. Z was given a printed name and address in large print on an 8½ × 11 sheet and asked to copy it directly below on the same sheet. Mr. Z omitted words on the left in the first two lines, but copied the third line correctly. His performance was very slow (Fig. 4).

Counting of Faces: Mr. Z was asked to count the people (37) in a picture and point to them as he counted. He missed twelve individuals on the left side. He counted two individuals twice. He counted in a random style, unable to maintain his place on a line, find the next line, or remember who he had or had not counted.

Bender: On the standard Bender Visual Motor Gestalt Test he showed the following difficulties: (a) spatial neglect—most of the figures are placed on the right side of the page, parts of the figures are missing, and (b) difficulties in spatial relations—lines are missing and points of intersection are vague (Figs. 6, 7).

Bisection of Lines: Mr. Z was asked to bisect a series of lines 10 and 15 cm long. He was also presented with a 10 cm bisected line and printed borders on a 5 × 8 index card and asked to copy it on a 8½ × 11 sheet of paper. This procedure was repeated for 10 cm and 15 cm lines without borders. He was also asked to draw his own line and bisect it. He performed as follows: (a) bisections were off the center toward the right, (b) the lines differed in size from the model, (c) free drawing was bisected off the center and tilted upward in a counter-clockwise fashion (Fig. 5).

Orientation to Time, Place, Person: Mr. Z was unable to tell time when he looked at

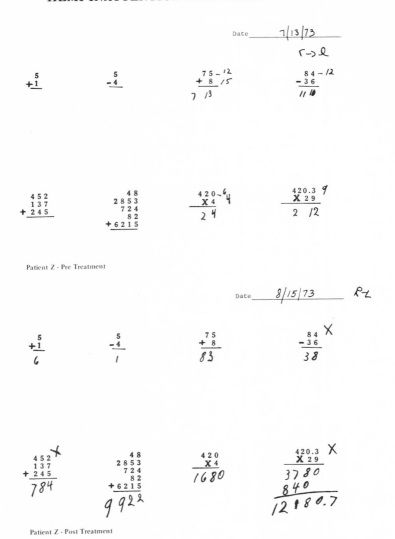

FIG. 2. Comparison of Patient Z performance pre- and post-treatment on wide range achievement arithmetic test.

a wristwatch and wall clock. He reported that he was unable to hold on to the two arrows on the face of the clock. He had no difficulty in telling the day of the week or the month and was able to tell how much time had elapsed since he ate breakfast, lunch, etc. He needed an attendant to take him to various classes because he could not find his way around the hospital. He was unable to give a description of the route from the testing room to his room, or from his room to the cafeteria. He forgot the examiner from day to day, and did not remember the testing room. These problems in orientation made the evaluation difficult and drawn out over time.

After 4 weeks of training, Mr. Z had learned to compensate for his spatial neglect and

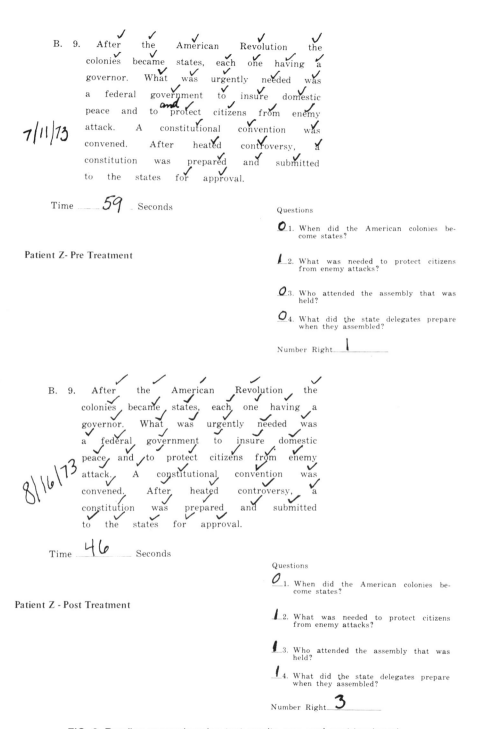

FIG. 3. Reading comprehension test results, pre- and post-treatment.

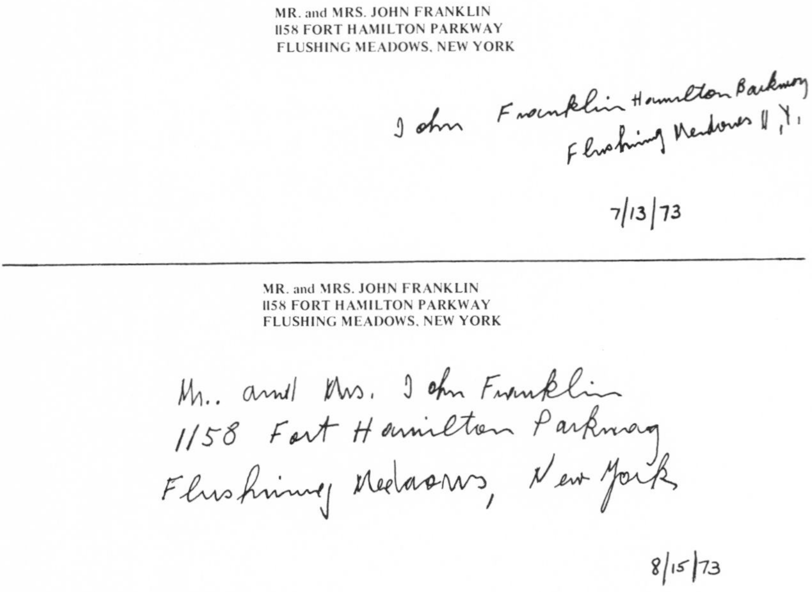

MR. and MRS. JOHN FRANKLIN
1158 FORT HAMILTON PARKWAY
FLUSHING MEADOWS. NEW YORK

John Fraunklin Hammilton Barkmay
Flushing Meadows 11, Y.

7/13/73

MR. and MRS. JOHN FRANKLIN
1158 FORT HAMILTON PARKWAY
FLUSHING MEADOWS. NEW YORK

Mr. and Mrs. John Franklin
1158 Fort Hamilton Parkmag
Flushinney Medaorvs, New York

8/15/73

FIG. 4. Copying an address test, pre- and post-treatment.

visual difficulties. He was reading books with regular print. Prior to training, he did not attend movies or watch television. After training, he frequently attended movies and watched television without difficulty. He returned with renewed interest to his old hobby of handicapping horses, and was anxious to make his first trip to the race track. He could once again read the racing form without problems. Mr. Z felt more independent now that he could tell the time, read his program card, and direct himself to his daily classes. There was no longer a need for an aide during meals, as there were no reports of his leaving out food located on the left side of his tray.

Follow-Up: Mr. Z was seen 1 year post training for follow-up progress report. He has not returned to work and spends most days with friends at home. He entertains himself by reading, watching TV, and handicapping horses. He frequently goes outside of his apartment by himself, occasionally to a park or a movie.

Mr. Z has maintained a high level of perceptual functioning. He performed on a par with his posttraining evaluation, when tested at this time. He reports that he has continued to perform scanning exercises and cancels out letters every day in his newspaper. He remembers training methods extremely well and appears oriented in all spheres.

Mr. A

Mr. A, a right-handed 64 year old businessman, had sustained a left hemiplegia secondary to a CVA. On admission to the rehabilitation program 2 months later, he was well-oriented, used a wheelchair and needed minimal assistance in activities of daily living. He exhibited a left hemianopsia and a decrease in sensation on the left side. He was placed on a typical rehabilitation program emphasizing physical and occupational therapy.

Mr. A had difficulty in shaving the left side of his face and combing his hair. Results

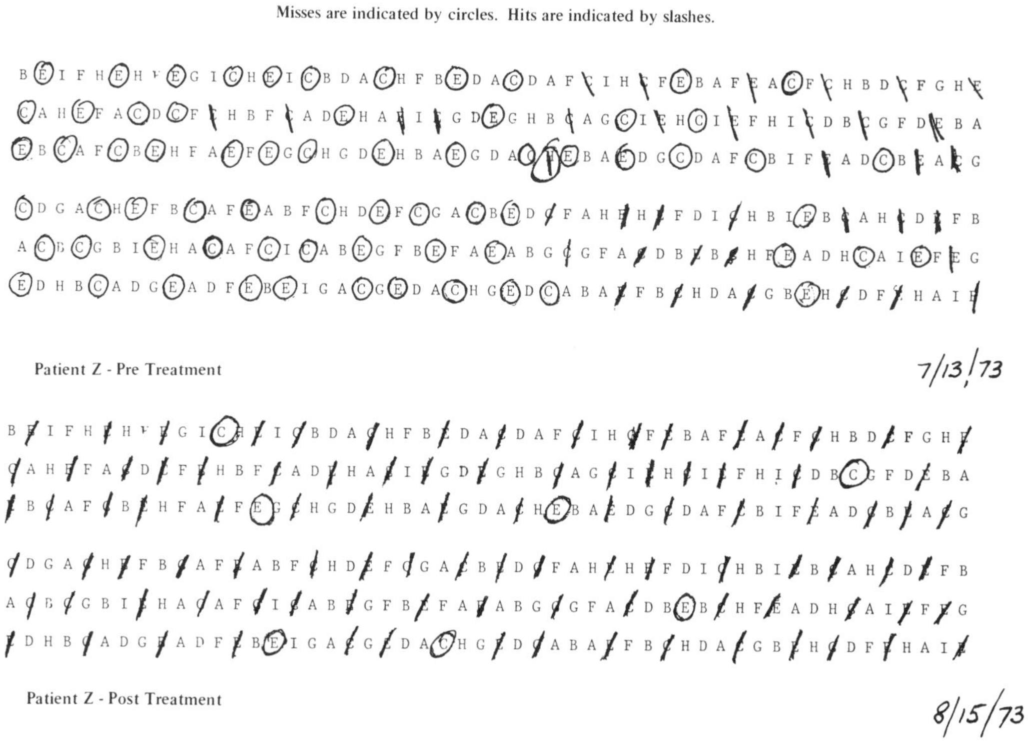

Misses are indicated by slashes. Hits are indicated by circles.

Patient Z - Pre Treatment

7/3/73

Patient Z - Post Treatment

8/15/73

FIG. 5. Cancellation of letters C and E, pre- and post-treatment.

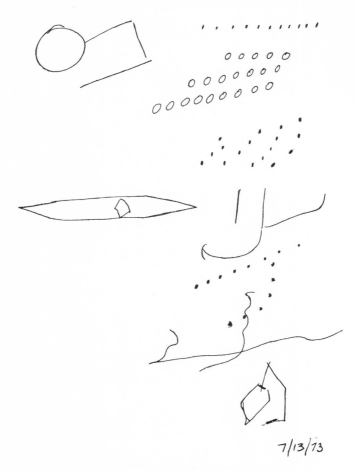

7/13/73

FIG. 6. Bender Visual Motor Gestalt Text, pre-treatment.

on initial testing indicated that he tended to leave out words on the left side when reading and omitted digits when performing simple arithmetical calculations. When his difficulties were pointed out to him, he did not appear concerned nor did he attempt to correct himself. He typically responded with statements such as, "I probably need new eyeglasses," "I am tired," "I was never an avid book reader." Generally, he showed little motivation in visual-perceptual training and claimed that he would learn to compensate for his difficulties without any special training.

He was retested on the same test battery a month later. His performance had deteriorated on most tests. For example, on the initial testing he copied the address correctly. On the second testing, he neglected part of the address. Similarly, there were no changes in his written calculation, nor did his scanning ability improve.

Functionally, in activities of daily living, there was no improvement. He still failed to shave his face on the left side, when wheeling himself he bumped against the wall, when eating he left out food on the left side and when reading he had difficulties in comprehension. He was then placed on a 1-month training program to improve his scanning.

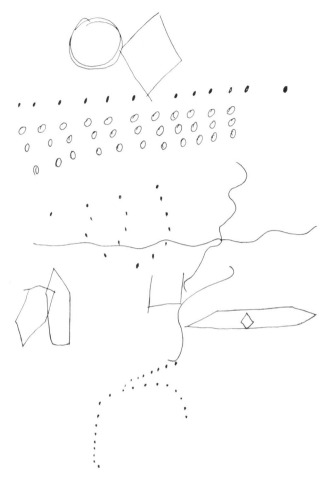

FIG. 7. Bender Visual Motor Gestalt Test, post-treatment.

Training: Despite efforts to induce an awareness of his visual spatial neglect and difficulty in organizing visual stimuli, he resisted participation in the training program. With the coaxing of his wife and physicians, he reluctantly agreed to attend classes. His attendance was spotty. However, as training proceeded and he began to compensate for his difficulties, he regularly attended the training sessions and asked for extra homework. He frequented the patient's library and used *The Reader's Digest* (large print). In addition, he became interested in watching television and took an active interest in his rehabilitation.

As he became aware of his neglect, Mr. A was no longer defensive of his visual-perceptual difficulties. For example, he was aware that something was amiss with his reading and that he could not comprehend the letters he received from his family, unless somebody read them to him.

Post-Testing: After 4 weeks of training, Fig. 8 (post-training) indicates that Mr. A had greatly compensated for his visual problems. His manner and style of executing the task

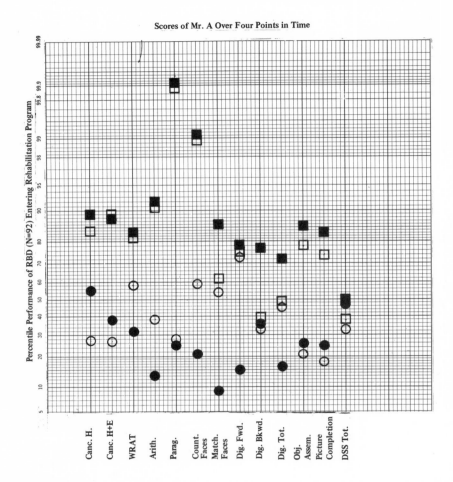

FIG. 8. Scores of Mr. A post-treatment. ○, pre control; ●, post control pre-training; □ post training; ■ follow-up.

also improved greatly. Prior to training he had approached tasks in an unsystematic system; after training, his style was orderly and careful.

On the cancellation tasks he improved greatly. He moved from the category of severely impaired to the category of mildly impaired. He was aware of errors and was also able to self correct. He also improved on copying an address and arithmetical calculation.

Comments: Mr. A's improved capacity to compensate for his visual-perceptual difficulties manifested itself on the visual-perceptual and academic tasks and was also evidenced in activities of daily living. He ventured to do things on his own and took an active part in social activities. He even started to plan to return to his business on a part-time basis.

Follow-Up: He was retested (fourth testing) 6 weeks post-training. As can be seen in Fig. 8, most of his performance remained stable and in some tasks he improved, e.g., calculation.

Conclusion

These cases indicate that it is possible to train RBD patients who suffer from hemi-inattention to compensate for their problems. Our clinical experience suggests that much of the disability can be related to a faulty set of habits that coexist with an actual disability imposed by neurologic defect. It is possible to teach people alternate ways of looking to compensate for the disabilities. The training consists of making the individual aware of the problem, forcing him to view stimuli systematically and repeating the procedure so that it becomes automatic.

ACKNOWLEDGMENTS

This study was supported in part under National Institutes of Health Grant No. SR01NS10236–05, Social and Rehabilitation Service, Department of Health, Education, and Welfare Grant No. RD-2666-P, and under the designation of New York University as a Rehabilitation Research and Training Center by Social and Rehabilitation Service, Department of Health, Education, and Welfare.

The authors would like to thank Ora Ezrachi, Wayne Gordon, and Louis Gerstman for their contributions to this paper.

REFERENCES

1. Bender, M. B. (1952): *Disorders in Perception with Particular Reference to the Phenomena of Extinction and Displacement.* Charles C Thomas, Springfield, Ill.
2. Bender, M. B., and Diamond, S. P. (1975): Sensory interaction effects and their relation to the organization of perceptual space. In: *The Nervous System. Vol. 3. Human Communication and its Disorders,* edited by D. B. Tower, pp. 393–402. Raven Press, New York.
3. Benton, A. L., and Van Allen, M. W. (1968): Impairment in facial recognition in patients with cerebral disease. *Cortex,* 4:344–358.
4. Diller, L., Ben-Yishay, Y., Gerstman, L., Goodkin, R., Gordon, W., Weinberg, J., et al. (1974): Rehabilitation Monograph 50, Studies in Cognition and Rehabilitation in Hemiplegia. NYU Medical Center, New York.
5. Diller, L., and Weinberg, J. (1970): Evidence for accident-prone behavior in hemiplegic patients. *Arch. Phys. Med. Rehabil.,* 51:353–363.
6. Gassel, M. M., and Williams, D. (1963): Visual function in patients with homonymous hemianopsia. *Brain,* 86:327.
7. Joynt, R. J., Benton, A. L., and Fogel, M. L. (1962): Behavioral and pathological correlates of motor impersistence. *Neurology,* 12:876–881.
8. Lawson, I. R. (1962): Visual-spatial neglect in lesions of the cerebral hemisphere. *Neurology,* 12:28–33.
9. Lorenze, E. J., and Cancro, R. (1962): Dysfunction in visual perception with hemiplegia: Its relation to activities of daily living. *Arch. Phys. Med. Rehabil.,* 43:514–517.
10. Luria, A. R. (1972): *The Man with a Shattered World.* Basic Books, New York.
11. Taylor, M. M., Schaeffer, J. N., Blumenthal, F. S., and Grissel, J. L. (1969): Controlled evaluation of perceptual and motor training therapy after stroke resulting in left hemiplegia. Final Report, Social and Rehabilitation Service, RD-2215-M. Department HEW, Washington, D.C.
12. Weinberg, J., Diller, L., Gerstman, L., and Schulman, P. (1972): Digit span in right and left hemiplegics. *J. Clin. Psychol.,* 28(3):361.
13. Weinberg, J., Diller, L., Gordon, W., Gerstman, L., Lieberman, A., Lakin, P., Hodges, G., and Ezrachi, O. (1977): Academic disabilities in acquired right brain damage. *Arch. Phys. Med. Rehabil. (Submitted for publication.)*

14. Weisbroth, S., Esibil, N., and Zuger, R. (1971): Factors in the vocational success of hemiplegic patients. *Arch. Phys. Med. Rehabil.*, 52:441–447.
15. Zane, M. D., and Goldman, H. (1966): Can responses to double simultaneous stimulation be improved in hemiplegic patients. *J. Nerv. Ment. Dis.*, 142:445–452.

DISCUSSION

Dr. Heilman: My first point is that I'm not really satisfied with the controls. Not treating a patient for one month is not a control. Patients do improve spontaneously and sometimes it takes over a month before the improvement begins. Secondly, have you compared groups, and how large a number of patients do you have?

Dr. Diller: With regard to the issues of controls: (a) although some patients with hemi-inattention might improve after the first 2 to 3 months, there is also a possibility that a number get worse because they have developed a poor gazing habit; (b) the largest gain of control patients falls below the median gain of the experimental patients; (c) follow-up data (1 year post of a sample of 20 patients—experimental and controls) indicates that the experimental group improves following treatment and may fall back slightly, but that the control group remains essentially the same as it did on leaving the rehabilitation program; (d) we have seen hemi-inattention patients several years post onset who respond to the procedure. With regard to the number of patients we have studied in formal experiments, we have conducted three independent studies. In these studies we used at least 30 controls with hemi-inattention. We might add that the control groups also receive some treatment. They receive routine occupational therapy designed to improve eye-hand skills in rehabilitation programs.

Mr. Weinberg: We now have about 40 patients.

Dr. Cohn: I have two questions. First, what about your failures? Then, you say that patients respond too fast. Isn't that, in part, a function of the way you present your material?

Dr. Diller: With regard to failures: (a) there are some patients who take longer than a month. Our treatment time is limited. In such cases, patients, at the end of the month, may show some improvement, but not enough to impact the criterion; (b) bilaterally damaged patients may have more difficulties than unilateral patients.

With regard to patients responding too fast, it must be noted that the materials are presented in a standard way. There is no great time pressure. One can slow the patient down by altering the standard presentation, e.g., asking the patient to verbalize as he performs. The problem of why a patient should respond too fast is interesting. In performing a cancellation task, left-brain damaged hemiplegics (most with aphasia) tend to respond too slowly. In right-brain damage, clinical observations suggest that the speed in cancellation is due to the patient's tendency to favor the right side of space. The patient acts as if he is "pulled" to the right. The speed may be related to task demands. In tasks such as block design, we have not noticed this.

Dr. Weinstein: This has been a most informative paper. When one attempts to alter a particular behavior, we learn new things about it, and these are what the authors have presented to us. I think they have shown, quite impressively, that some aspects of the behavior of hemi-inattentive patients are subject to modification. Another major feature is that it takes up the very significant role of motivation in the genesis and maintenance of hemi-inattention.

There are several questions and issues that can be raised. The first concerns the definition of hemi-inattention. Should we include such disturbances as disorientation for time, dressing apraxia, poor calculation, errors in dialing a telephone and making sense of a television show under the rubric of hemi-neglect? It is true that we do find these problems in our hemi-inattentive patients, but they are far more common in patients who do not manifest hemi-neglect. Also, most patients with hemi-neglect do not have dressing apraxia and topographical disorientation, even though right parietal lobe lesions are common.

Now what is the mechanism whereby your patients improve? I noticed that Patients A and Z not only had significantly less neglect after their training, but improved in a wide variety of tasks. Patient Z showed a spectacular improvement in reading and matching faces. Surprisingly, he showed much less improvement in counting faces, a task that I would suppose to be more closely related to hemi-inattention than matching faces. This casts some doubt on the thesis that you are specifically treating hemi-inattention.

I was interested in the statement that Mr. Z, your first patient, became very depressed because of the problems created by his neglect of his left side, causing him to feel deprived and useless. I wonder if one could say, with as much justification, that his marked mood change and apathy contributed to the neglect. I would think that there is some kind of a reciprocal interaction. We do know that so-called psychological factors do influence hemi-inattention. I recall the case of a man who, having recovered from a ruptured aneurysm, was called down to the Bureau of Internal Revenue to explain why he hadn't paid his taxes. On ordinary clinical examination, his left hemi-inattention was extremely mild. However, he was almost run over when he failed to notice a truck coming from his left while crossing the street. Inside the building he was almost arrested when he entered a ladies room after having misread the sign WOMEN as MEN. It seems to me that here the stress temporarily duplicated the effects of the previously more severe brain damage.

I would emphasize, again, the selective, symbolic, motivational factors of conspicuous hemi-neglect. In the paper by Ian Lawson, cited by Dr. Diller and Mr. Weinberg, the patient's reading improved after training, but she still showed hemi-inattention in her drawings. Does Dr. Diller feel that the "hard core" features of hemi-inattention, namely eye shift and extinction on DSS, can be modified by training? It is these that are the most enduring in spontaneous recovery.

Dr. Diller: With regard to the definition of hemi-inattention: (a) all the phenomena we have cited are visually contingent and therefore vulnerable to disturbances in hemi-inattention. For example, by disturbance in time we mean telling time from a clock or reading a program card. We refer to written as opposed to aural arithmetic. We recognize that many behaviors, e.g., dialing a telephone, are complex and may be failed by different patients for different reasons. Difficulties here might occur in the absence of hemi-inattention; (b) we have not touched on perceptual problems that may overlay hemi-inattention or the problems presented in right-brain damage without hemi-inattention. In repeated factor analysis, which we have conducted with right-brain-damaged patients, hemi-inattention emerges as one factor underlying skills structure. Following treatment, there is a shift in the organization of skills; (c) our sample is composed largely of hemiparetics and hemiplegics. Whether hemi-inattention in the absence of hemiplegia has a different pattern we can't say; (d) the behaviors we cited were part of a pattern, but need not be present in every case.

With regard to the mechanism of the improvement, several comments: (a) Patient Z did indeed show improvement in counting faces. On a picture containing 37 faces, he originally counted 18 correct. Following treatment he counted 30. However, the gain did not show because of the distribution of the test scores. On this particular task the control group also improved; (b) The patient's improvement could also be seen in other ways than total number correct. In the precondition, the patient counted only 1 of 12 figures on the left side of the page. He also counted a figure on the right twice. In the postcondition, the patient counted the left faces correctly. The errors were due to the omission of an entire single row of faces.

Dr. Weinstein's comment points up an interesting fact. Patients learn new habits as a result of the training. These habits still differ from the way normal people approach a task and may not be adequate for certain situations, e.g., task completion, stress, fatigue. The interplay of hemi-inattention and motivational states does exist and is, therefore, important.

We believe that the hard core features of hemi-inattention, such as eye shift and extinction on DSS, can indeed be modified. Our observations on eye shift are based on a gross clinical level. We hope to explore this, using more refined methods of observing eye movements. With regard to DSS phenomena, particularly the face-hand test, the studies of Zane and Goldman merely indicate that one can coach a patient to perform on a given task. However, this need not indicate that a change in underlying skills has occurred. We have some evidence that such changes can occur. However, the training program must be enriched to encompass the utilization of the body in space and not be confined to visual scanning. Our studies suggest that training in visual scanning can be an underlying substrate for training in a variety of areas related to phenomena associated with extinction, body image, and visual perception. The interesting problem here is to what skills does training generalize? If one wants to widen the network of skills, then one must widen the training. Scanning training is no panacea. It does open the patient to permit us to (a) examine other perceptual behaviors once the problem in scanning is overcome, and (b) examine the substructures involved in perception.

Dr. Diamond: Thank you, Dr. Diller. I hope that you have convinced the skeptics.

Advances in Neurology, Vol. 18, edited by E. A.
Weinstein and R. P. Friedland. Raven Press,
New York © 1977.

Manifestations and Implications of Shifting Hemi-Inattention in Commissurotomy Patients

Jerre Levy

Department of Psychology, University of Pennsylvania, Philadelphia, Pennsylvania 19174

During the past several years, a great deal of attention has been focused on the nature of the specialized abilities of the left and right cerebral hemispheres. Dramatic differences in the cognitive capacities of the two sides of the brain have been revealed with particular clarity in commissurotomy patients. The left hemisphere has been shown to surpass the right, not only in language expression (12), but also in language comprehension (17), in pattern recognition for patterns whose features are not spatially constrained (8), and in phonetic imaging, even when neither speech perception nor expression is required (6). The right hemisphere, in contrast, is superior to the left in three-dimensional visualization, the recognition of faces and nonsense shapes, and imagistic encoding (5).

The above capacity differences of the hemispheres have been seen with a variety of experimental paradigms and are assumed to reflect differences in the underlying neuroanatomical structures on the left and right (3,4,15,16). However, there also appear to be differences in the dynamic properties of the cerebral hemispheres that change with situational variables, specifically, differences in the extent to which one or the other side of the brain is aroused and attentive.

Using bilateral hemispheric stimulation in commissurotomy patients, Levy et al. (8) and Levy and Trevarthen (6,7) found that, under some conditions, the right hemisphere assumed control of behavior, whereas under other conditions, the left hemisphere did so. Furthermore, whenever one half-brain gained control of the response, it appeared as if the other half were totally unaware that it had been presented with a stimulus. Levy et al. (8) concluded that, if the required response was one of which either hemisphere was capable, then neither the nature of the stimulus nor the nature of the response determined hemispheric dominance for a task, but rather hemispheric control was a function of the cognitive processing demands. They pointed out that there could be a positive, negative, or zero correlation between the relative performance abilities of the hemispheres and the relative tendencies to take control of behavior. In other words, it was found that although one side of the brain might have been no better or even worse than the other in some cognitive task, it, nevertheless, might selectively attempt cognitive processing and control of the behavioral response.

This conclusion led Levy and Trevarthen (7) to postulate that the human cerebral hemispheres were not only specialized in cognitive ability but also with respect to intentions to act, and that the neural substrates mediating these two specializations were, to a certain extent, independent. They reasoned that if this were so, it was possible for the "wrong" hemisphere to take control of behavior, i.e., the hemisphere that is less adept at solving the problem at hand.

In order to investigate this possibility, a test was designed that permitted either hemisphere to respond to its stimulus and in which the response could either be based on the recognition of a visual similarity or a conceptual similarity between the stimulus and choice. Examples of stimuli and choice pictures are shown in Fig. 1. The left half of one picture was joined to the right half of another and the resultant chimera was tachistoscopically projected so that the midline of the stimulus coincided with the patient's fixation point. Under these conditions, as Levy et al. (8) and Trevarthen and Kinsbourne (14) showed previously, each hemisphere of the commissurotomy patient effects a perceptual completion of the half-stimulus it receives. Patients were instructed that they would see "a picture in the machine" and that they were to point to a picture, from among an array in free vision, that was similar in some way to the one briefly exposed.

A first test was administered to only one patient, N.G., with ambiguous instructions as to the strategy of matching. N.G. was told to "pick the one which is like,

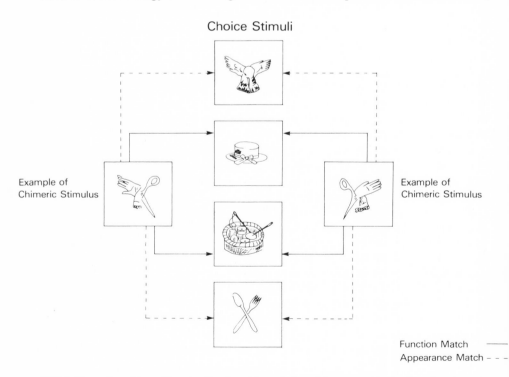

FIG. 1. Examples of two chimeric stimuli and four choice pictures used in the Function-Appearance Matching Test.

goes with, or is similar in some way to what you see." The purpose of this test was to confirm that the right and left hemispheres, when they responded under these conditions, would match according to visual and conceptual similarity, respectively.

This expectation was completely confirmed. On some trials, the patient matched the stimulus seen by the right hemisphere, and, when she did so, the match was based on visual similarity. On other trials, the left-hemisphere stimulus was matched, and, when this occurred, the match was based on a functional categorization.

The results of the test confirm our understanding of hemispheric specialization and suggest, also, that there are internal, time-variant processes that shift the balance of arousal between the hemispheres. Specifically, it appears that whichever hemisphere happens to have the activation advantage at the time a stimulus is presented becomes even further aroused, processes its input, and gains access to the final common path. We never saw an instance in which N.G. pointed to two choices, or any evidence that the nonresponding hemisphere was disturbed by the choice made. It was as if the nonresponding hemisphere were totally blind for the contralateral visual field. Though this hemi-inattention shifted throughout the trials from one to the other visual half-field, it appeared to have the same characteristics as hemi-inattention resulting from unilateral cortical lesions. It differed only in that the hemi-inattention was unstable with respect to the side on which it occurred.

We reasoned that external demands ought to be able to influence the selective activation of the hemispheres but that such demands would, on occasion, be inconsistent with the internal state. If so, it could be expected that dissociations would occur such that task instructions might elicit the appropriate matching strategy without arousing the hemisphere specialized for it, or might arouse the appropriate hemisphere but fail to induce its specialized matching strategy. If such dissociations did, in fact, occur, it would be hard to doubt that the neural processes responsible for ability differences in the hemispheres were separate from those mediating selective activation.

A second test was run on four patients, including N.G., but each patient was run under two conditions. Under one condition, the patient was instructed to "pick the one which *looks* similar to what you see" (appearance instruction), and under the other condition to "pick the one which *goes* with or that you would *use* with what you see" (function instruction).

Each of the four patients displayed a different pattern of results, summarized in Fig. 2. In all except one, dissociations occurred. Although appearance and function instructions asymmetrically produced right- and left-hemisphere responses, respectively, in all four patients and elicited the appropriate matching strategy in three, the hemisphere and strategy did not necessarily occur together. As may be seen in Fig. 2, although patient C.C. showed appropriate shifts in hemispheric control with shifting instructions, he always matched according to visual similarity. N.G., on this test, responded with the left hemisphere and with

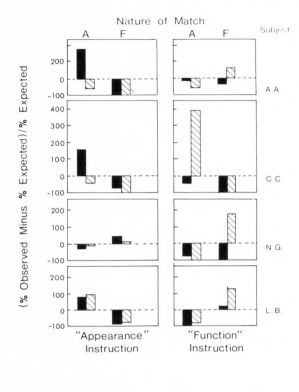

FIG. 2. Summary of the performance of four split-brain patients under two instructional conditions on the Function-Appearance Matching Test. A = appearance match, F = function match. (Reprinted with permission from reference 7: Copyright 1976 by the American Psychological Association.)

conceptual matches in response to function instructions, but continued, to some extent, to make conceptual matches in response to appearance instructions and allocated her responses fairly evenly between the hemispheres. L.B. displayed consistent matches according to task instructions but did not shift to complete right-hemisphere control under appearance instructions. Only A.A. showed consistent shifts in both hemispheric control and in strategy of matching under both sets of instructions.

In these tests, patients were required to point to their choices with the *right* hand with appearance instructions and with the *left* hand under function instructions. This was done as a conservative technique, to assure that hemispheric control would not be induced by the use of the contralateral hand. However, it is quite possible that this requirement increased the probability of dissociations by tending to bias the task-inappropriate hemisphere that was contralateral to the pointing hand.

Evidence that this is so was obtained in a subsequent set of trials with L.B. In an attempt to break the hold that the left hemisphere seemed to have on behavior (see Fig. 2), we ran L.B. under appearance instructions with left-hand pointing. In contrast to his previous trials with right-hand pointing, the right hemisphere assumed control of behavior and responded on 100% of trials. After providing this "reinforcement" to the right hemisphere, L.B. was switched back to right-hand pointing under appearance instructions and the right hemisphere maintained complete control. A final run of trials under function instructions were given with left-hand pointing, and, as on earlier trials under these conditions, the left hemisphere took control of all responses. Thus, the balance of activation between the two sides of the brain may be shifted by switching the responding hand, and the balance may be preserved even when the responding hand is switched back.

The results of the preceding studies have led us to propose that a hemisphere takes control of processing and behavior in accordance with what it *thinks* it can do, and only indirectly in accordance with its actual abilities. We have suggested that task instructions are processed and analyzed by both the left and right cerebral cortices; descending impulses are, in consequence, directed into brainstem regions and, in particular, into the midbrain reticular system, where they elicit ipsilateral, ascending, activating impulses and induce asymmetric arousal of the hemispheres. In the intact brain, it would be expected that the neocortical commissures would participate in controlling and maintaining adaptive, asymmetric activation in accordance with cognitive demands. The dissociations we observed would be, in part, due to the depletion of this higher level control, although recent studies of Gur, Gur, and Harris (2) demonstrate conclusively that, under conditions of stress, the normal, intact brain displays similar dissociations.

The positive feedback interaction between a hemisphere and the brainstem in controlling attention into the two visual half-fields is elegantly demonstrated in Sprague's experiment with cats (13). Ablation of the striate cortex on one side produced total blindness for the contralateral field. When, however, the superior colliculus contralateral to the lesioned cortex was also ablated, vision was restored to both visual half-fields. It seems clear that the hemi-inattention produced by the cortical lesion resulted from an imbalance in activation to the two sides of the brain, an imbalance that was rectified by the subsequent unilateral destruction of the superior colliculus on the opposite side. Our studies with split-brain patients rather strongly suggest that in people, as in cats, hemi-inattention is a direct consequence of deficient arousal in one hemisphere as compared with the other, a deficiency that is proximally the result of an insufficiency of activating impulses from brainstem regions, but that is ultimately the result of an inadequacy in the cortex itself in eliciting arousal. Given our results with these patients and the fact that external factors are effective in shifting the balance of attention, there is a firm theoretical ground for believing that various therapies could be devised for correcting hemi-inattention in unilaterally brain-damaged patients.

Although it is probably the case that the maximum absolute level of arousal of which a damaged hemisphere is capable is depressed relative to an intact brain, it is likely that lateralized attentional deficits are more a function of the degree of imbalance of attention in the two sides of the brain than of the actual magnitude of arousal potential in the injured hemisphere. The correction of hemi-inattention would seem to require both an induction of maximal possible arousal in the damaged side of the brain, as well as the production of inhibition in the intact side. The achievement of the latter end would appear to be at least as important as the achievement of the former in alleviating hemi-inattention.

It is suggested that the functional deficits that are correlated with any type of cortical damage are caused, not so much by the destruction of a region in which a function is localized, but rather by the fact that the ease with which a finely tuned, unique, spatiotemporal pattern of activation and inhibition, involving the entire cerebrum and essential for the functional integrity of a given behavioral system, has been enormously decreased by the lesion in question. Quite obviously, a lesion may not only impose difficulties in the achievement of the essential neural pattern but may make it totally impossible. Nevertheless, the efficacy of both time and therapy in effecting at least a partial recovery of function following cortical damage (a recovery, moreover, for which little explanation has been given) suggests that in many, if not most, cases the restoration is not impossible even though it may be extremely difficult to restore in the face of cerebral damage.

The mammalian brain, almost by definition, is an organ of extreme plasticity in terms of the means available to it to achieve some end. Unlike the brains of lower animals in which systems are tightly wired, each subsystem of the mammalian brain, and particularly of the human brain, has widespread access, through a multiplicity of pathways, to other subsystems in the neural network. Learning itself is quite probably the changing of thresholds of access among various regions of the central nervous system, and, if the view of the brain-behavior relationship being emphasized here is correct, if, in other words, it is the dynamics of neural function rather than the static presence or absence of some piece of cortical tissue per se that determine behavioral adaptation, a firm theoretical foundation is provided for neuropsychological therapy and a number of therapeutic techniques could be devised based on this conception.

Sperry has proposed, in his recent publications, that human beings, in a very real sense, are free agents; that the overall spatiotemporal pattern of neural activity that is consciousness, involving all cortical regions and in interaction with the brainstem, has causal control over lower level, less holistic systems; that human beings can and do behave in accordance with their conscious intentions (9–11). What is meant by this proposal is simply that the emergent property of higher level neural activity, which is experienced as consciousness, possesses its own operational characteristics that constrain and control the lower level constituents, in the same way that the organizational properties of any organ constrain and control the activities of its cells. Of importance in the conception is the idea that the critical operational characteristics do not depend on a single, unique, causal chain but may be achieved by any number of underlying interactions. Though some have attributed to Sperry's conceptualization both mysticism and dualism (1), careful reading of his papers makes clear that his position represents a generalization to the realm of consciousness of the emergent functions always arising from material organization. Just as liquidity may arise from the interactions of any number and kinds of molecules, or sphericality may describe a property of objects regardless of the elements of which they are composed, so may characteristics of consciousness, such as pain, arise from a multitude of interactions among subpatterns of neural activity. In the presence of a brain lesion, it may be difficult to achieve some spatiotemporal pattern of neural activity necessary for functional integrity, but if Sperry's conception is correct, then as long as consciousness is present at all, there is some finite probability that the critical pattern features of some behavioral system can, with time, effort, and therapy, be regained.

REFERENCES

1. Bindra, D. (1970): The problem of subjective experience: Puzzlement on reading R. W. Sperry's "A modified concept of consciousness." *Psychol. Rev.,* 77:581–584.
2. Gur, R. E., Gur, R. C., and Harris, L. J. (1975): Hemispheric activation, as measured by the subjects' conjugate lateral eye movements, is influenced by experimenter location. *Neuropsychologia,* 13:35–44.
3. LeMay, M., and Culebras, A. (1972): Human brain—morphologic differences in the hemispheres demonstrable by carotid arteriography. *N. Engl. J. Med.,* 287:168–170.
4. Levitsky, W., and Geschwind, N. (1968): Human brain: Left-right asymmetries in temporal speech region. *Science,* 161:186–187.
5. Levy, J. (1974): Psychobiological implications of bilateral asymmetry. In: *Hemisphere Function in the Human Brain,* edited by S. Dimond and J. G. Beaumont. Paul Elek, London.
6. Levy, J., and Trevarthen, C. (1977): Perceptual, semantic, and phonetic aspects of elementary language processes in split-brain patients. *Brain (In press.)*
7. Levy, J., and Trevarthen, C. (1976): Meta-control of hemispheric function in human split-brain patients. *J. Exp. Psychol.: Hum. Percept. Perform.,* 2:299–312.
8. Levy, J., Trevarthen, C., and Sperry, R. W. (1972): Perception of bilateral chimeric figures following hemispheric deconnection. *Brain,* 95:61–78.
9. Sperry, R. W. (1969): A modified concept of consciousness. *Psychol. Rev.,* 76:532–536.
10. Sperry, R. W. (1970): An objective approach to subjective experience: Further explanation of a hypothesis. *Psychol. Rev.,* 77:585–590.
11. Sperry, R. W. (1974): Mental phenomena as causal determinants in brain function. In: *Mind and Brain: Philosophic and Scientific Strategies,* edited by F. O. Schmitt and F. G. Worden. MIT Press, Cambridge, Mass.
12. Sperry, R. W., Gazzaniga, M. S., and Bogen, J. E. (1969): Interhemispheric relationships: The neocortical commissures; syndromes of hemisphere disconnection. In: *Handbook of Clinical Neurology, IV,* edited by P. J. Vinken and G. W. Bruyn. North Holland, Amsterdam.
13. Sprague, J. M. (1966): Interaction of cortex and superior colliculus in mediation of visually guided behavior in the cat. *Science,* 153:1544–1547.
14. Trevarthen, C., and Kinsbourne, M. (1974): Perceptual completion of words and figures by commissurotomy patients. *(Unpublished material.)*
15. Wada, J., Clarke, R., and Hamm, A. (1975): Cerebral hemispheric asymmetry in humans. Cortical speech zones in 100 adult and 100 infant brains. *Arch. Neurol.,* 32:239–246.

16. Witelson, S. F., and Pallie, W. (1973): Left hemisphere specialization for language in the newborn: Neuroanatomical evidence of asymmetry. *Brain,* 96:641–647.
17. Zaidel, E. (1976): Auditory vocabulary in the right hemisphere following brain bisection and hemidecortication. *Cortex,* 12:191–211.

DISCUSSION

Dr. Heilman: I have a question for Dr. Levy. I was wondering, in your patients with chimeric stimuli, did the patients, in their normal behavior, report anything or did you see anything that would make you think that in their day-to-day activities they had problems in identification?

Dr. Levy: Yes, I believe so. A number of these patients reported—that is their left hemispheres reported—that their attention span was too short. Apparently they would be reading normally and all of a sudden they would no longer be reading. I suspect that the corpus callosum plays a major role in maintaining attention in one hemisphere, adaptively, and will only switch attention to the other hemisphere when there's a reason for it. In the absence of the corpus callosum, I get the impression that the left hemisphere might be turned on, as it were, while the patients are reading. Suddenly, because there's a lack of higher level control mediated by the callosum, the right hemisphere may be activated, disrupting the ongoing cognitive activity of the left hemisphere. In addition, there appears to be a splitting in certain kinds of memory traces.

When I was running the face tests, one of the patients said to me, "How is Dr. Sperry? I haven't seen Dr. Sperry in a long time." I said, "He's fine, N. . . .", to which she responded, "Tell him I said hello when you see him." At this point she decided to get some water. She walked out of the laboratory into the hallway, passing Dr. Sperry on her way to the water fountain. They smiled at each other without speaking and, after getting her water, N. . . . returned to the laboratory and said, "Who was that man out in the hall that I just passed? He looked vaguely familiar, but I don't know who he is." This was about two minutes after talking about Sperry, whom she had known by this time for five years. It was as if the left hemisphere had encoded the memory of Sperry in ways not having to do with what his face looked like. There was a splitting of memory traces, I believe.

Dr. Weinstein: Dr. Levy, you cite an interesting incident, but I wonder about your explanation. According to D. Zaidel and Sperry, their callosally sectioned patients did have memory loss. I recall that some of them did not remember where they had parked their cars. My impression is that this memory loss is due to injury at surgery to the underlying fornix and cingulate area, important structures for memory function. Dr. Gazzaniga told me recently that his new series of patients who have had callosal sections at Dartmouth do not have such memory loss. With due respect for Dr. Joseph Bogen, I think that the difference is in the surgery.

Dr. Levy: Again, my interpretation of this kind of memory loss is a split of different kinds of memories that are being laid down here. I am not convinced there is a global loss in memory here. There *appears* to be a global loss because certain kinds of memories depend on the retrieval of two kinds of memories, separately encoded in the two hemispheres. In the absence of the neocortical commissures, the two kinds of memory traces cannot be integrated.

Dr. Weinstein: I would agree with Dr. Levy that one would not expect a global memory loss. But, with lesions in the fornix and other limbic structures, one does get selective amnesia, such as occurred between your patient and Dr. Sperry. It is common for such a patient to do well on a standard memory scale and not be able to remember having seen the examiner before or recall the name of the hospital, or remember what the problem was that brought him to the hospital.

I think the issue is important to our understanding of unilateral neglect, as we have seen how selective the patient can be in forgetting what is happening on the affected side. I think that Dr. Heilman and I have both made the point that severe hemi-neglect depends on a limbic lesion.

Dr. Heilman: Let me answer that question, also, and let me ask a question about it. First of all, we did some callosal sections in monkeys to see what effect it would have on unilateral neglect syndrome, and it's very difficult to get to the corpus callosum without hitting the cingulate gyrus. Now, I don't know, this is in a monkey and I haven't seen any human callosal cuts, but I would imagine they would probably injure the cingulate gyrus, also, and it is part of the Papez circuit and one can't help wondering if this involves memory.

The other thing is that the fornix does travel quite close by, and we have some good evidence now, which I won't get into, that fornicotomy—fornicotomy-defornication —anyway, cutting the fornix—does produce an amnestic state very similar to temporal lobectomy. I think we have very good evidence about that.

Dr. Weinstein: I'd like to ask Dr. Levy about those reports by Eran Zaidel and Michael Gazzaniga about patients who did not report they saw a stimulus in the visual field, but who showed an appropriate emotional response. Gazzaniga has a movie in which sexy pictures are flashed into the left visual field. While the patient denied seeing anything, her giggle was unmistakable. This is a classical example of hemi-neglect.

Now, are these occasional observations that may happen once in a while in one of the patients, or is it a regular feature? If it is, it would be an extremely important thing in that the referential meaning of something is lost, but the emotional significance is preserved.

Dr. Levy: I think what occurs in these cases is simply the following: An emotionally arousing stimulus is projected to the right hemisphere, and the right hemisphere, being a human brain, gets an emotional reaction. The emotional reaction has bodily concomitants to it, for example, giggling and blushing responses generated by the right hemisphere. Now, surely the left hemisphere is aware of the giggling, and when the investigator says, "What are you giggling about?", the left hemisphere has to justify this rather strange behavior. The comments one gets out of the left hemisphere under these conditions are justifications for quite correctly observed evidence of some sort of emotional state. I see nothing very mysterious in the process.

In work with split-brain animals in which learning by one or the other hemisphere has been reinforced by unilateral electrical stimulation of the medial forebrain bundle, it has been found that such stimulation reinforces learning only when it is ipsilateral to the side of visual stimulus input. On the basis of such findings, I conclude that affective states do not spread from one hemisphere to the other, except by the secondary means of having bodily reactions, which the left hemisphere picks up. I realize that this conclusion contrasts with that of Gazzaniga, as he stated it in his original article, but I have never agreed with his position on this issue.

Dr. Pasik: Dr. Levy, in your testing situation you are ruling out the potential role of eye movements because of your tachistoscopic exposure. I should like you to comment on the possibility that you may not be obviating their role completely. It is conceivable that one hemisphere may, in fact, "issue the command" to move the eyes, and, although the actual execution of the movements occurs when the stimuli have already disappeared, the visual system may be getting some information about the direction of the eventual ocular deviations.

Dr. Levy: I agree with you completely on this. In fact, various studies with normals in psychology looking at what happens with tachistoscopic presentation do indicate that there is a cognitive scanning, as it were, of iconic images of stimuli, even though the eyes are not actually moving. I am quite certain that the same thing is occurring in the split-brain patient. The actual eye movement is simply delayed until after the stimulus has disappeared. An attentional scan was quite probably occurring that had the same processing effect on attention as if there had been an actual scan. However, an attentional scan of an iconic image, unlike an actual scan of a real stimulus, cannot project a stimulus to the left or right of a fixation point, to the ipsilateral hemisphere.

Dr. Cohn: In your pictures of the eyeball movements, that was a DC recording you had, I notice, and also you had these oscillatory, something like microsaccades. Were they microsaccades or was that just noise?

Dr. Levy: I think that was just noise.

Dr. Cohn: Well, it was a funny noise.

Dr. Levy: I am no expert in electrooculograms, so if you believe the "noise" represents microsaccades, I am perfectly willing to yield to your judgment. I do not know how to determine from the polygraph output just what the oscillations might mean.

Advances in Neurology, Vol. 18, edited by E. A. Weinstein and R. P. Friedland. Raven Press, New York © 1977.

Mechanisms Underlying the Unilateral Neglect Syndrome

Kenneth M. Heilman and Robert T. Watson

Department of Neurology, College of Medicine, University of Florida, and Veterans Administration Hospital, Gainesville, Florida 32610

We should like to define the neglect syndrome as a unilateral defect in the orienting response. During the acute stage, one sees a complete loss of the orienting reflex to the side contralateral to the lesion. The patient, therefore, ignores all contralateral sensory stimuli and demonstrates a poverty of movement. This stage has been termed "unilateral neglect," also called "hemi-neglect" and "hemi-inattention." Because the patient is unable to orient to the contralateral field, he may orient to the ipsilateral side even when stimuli are applied contralaterally. This behavior is similar to what has been termed "allesthesia" (53). As the patient recovers, he may be capable of orienting to the contralateral field when unilateral stimuli are applied to the contralateral side. The orienting response to the contralateral field, however, is weaker than that to the ipsilateral side; and, when a patient is given bilateral simultaneous stimulation, he orients only to the normal side. This behavior has been termed "extinction to simultaneous stimulation" (5).

Since patients with neglect, allesthesia, and extinction exhibit different behavior, there can be little doubt that the pathophysiology underlying each of these behavioral aberrations is different. Before discussing these differences, however, we should look at some of the mechanisms proposed to explain why there is a disturbance of the orienting reflex in all three of these stages.

In general, four different general theories have been used to explain the neglect syndrome: (a) a perceptual defect (e.g., visuospatial agnosia, amorphosynthesis), (b) a sensory defect, (c) an attention-arousal defect, and (d) a defect in interhemispheric inhibition.

PERCEPTUAL HYPOTHESES

Visuospatial Agnosia

Brain (11) believed that the parietal lobe contained the body schema. Since spatial perception is also mediated by the parietal lobe, with parietal lesions, a patient fails to recognize not only half of his body but also half of space. Subsequently, Paterson and Zangwill (55) and McFie, Piercy, and Zangwill (48) also demonstrated that patients with right parietal dysfunction had visuospatial disorders associated with neglect. Both groups recognized that neglect could not completely explain the visuospatial disorder, but they did not mention whether the visuospatial disorder could explain neglect.

Amorphosynthesis

Denny-Brown, Meyer, and Horenstein (18) and Denny-Brown and Banker (17) proposed that the disorder underlying the neglect syndrome was not a defect of spatial relationships or body image as had been previously suggested, but rather was a defect in spatial perception. Neglect in man is most frequently associated with parietal dysfunction (11,14,15,18). Denny-Brown and associates (18) thought that the parietal lobes were important in cortical sensation and the phenomenon of tactile inattention belonged to the whole class of cortical disorders of sensation: ". . . a loss of finer discrimination . . . an inability to synthesize more than a few properties of a sensory stimulus and a disturbance of synthesis of multiple sensory stimuli." They also believed that sensory synthesis was important in spatial summation (morphosynthesis) and the behavioral defect seen in the neglect syndrome was a defect in sensory synthesis (i.e., amorphosynthesis).

DEAFFERENTATION HYPOTHESES

Battersby, Bender, and Pollack (3) postulated that the neglect syndrome was produced by both a defect in sensation and an altered mental status. The observations of Sprague, Chambers, and Stellar (64) gave support to the Battersby group's hypothesis. Sprague and co-workers interrupted the lateral portion of the mesencephalon and induced neglect. Since the lateral regions of the mesencephalon contain ascending sensory pathways, they concluded that neglect was due to a loss of sensory input to the neocortex. More recently, Eidelberg and Schwartz (20) proposed a similar hypothesis, namely that neglect is a passive phenomenon caused by asymmetrical sensory input into the two hemispheres or by an asymmetry of functional mass of the areas concerned with somatic sensation.

ATTENTIONAL HYPOTHESES

Some of the first references in the literature (35–37) referred to defects of attention. Poppelreuter (56) introduced the word "inattention" to refer to the neglect syndrome. Brain (11) and Critchley (14) were also strong proponents of this view. Bender and Furlow (6,7), however, challenged the attentional theory; they felt that inattention could not be important in the pathophysiology of the syndrome, because causing the patient to "concentrate" on the neglected side did not alter the deficit.

Recently, Heilman and Valenstein (31) and Watson and associates (72) have again postulated an attention-arousal hypothesis. It has been demonstrated that patients with unilateral neglect most often have their dysfunction in the inferior parietal lobule (14,30,32). The inferior parietal lobule appears to be a secondary association area. The primary sensory areas (i.e., auditory, visual, somesthetic) project to their own association areas, and each of these association areas projects to the inferior parietal lobule (54). Experimental lesions restricted to this region can produce multimodal neglect in monkeys (27). By recording cellular electrical activity, Yin and colleagues (78) demonstrated that there were neurons in these inferior parietal lobules that discharged before the onset of an orienting response to visual stimuli. Stimuli in the contralateral field appeared to be most effective in eliciting these responses. There also appeared to be neurons in the same area that responded to auditory stimuli. Onset of certain tones appeared not only to excite certain cells but also to influence the usual cell response to a visual stimulus (16).

Pandya and Kuypers (54) have also shown that auditory, visual, and somesthetic association areas project to the dorsolateral frontal lobe. The inferior parietal lobe also projects to the dorsolateral frontal lobe. Lesions in this tertiary association area also produce neglect in animals (40,76) and in man (31).

Heilman and Valenstein (31) also noted that several patients with unilateral neglect had discrete lesions in the cingulate gyrus. To confirm the clinical observations, Watson and associates (72) demonstrated that, in primates, discrete unilateral lesions in the anterior cingulate gyrus produce unilateral neglect. Interestingly, Pandya and Kuypers (54) showed that the dorsolateral frontal lobe projects to the cingulate gyrus. Because unilateral neglect could be produced outside of the traditional primary sensory and sensory association areas, Heilman and Valenstein (31) and Watson and co-workers (72) felt that the sensory and perceptual hypothesis, although perhaps a first-order explanation, could not serve as a unifying concept.

Moruzzi and Magoun (50) showed that the reticular formation is important in mediation of the orienting response. Since neglect appeared to be a defect in the orienting response, Heilman and Valenstein (31) and Watson and associates (72) postulated that unilateral neglect was a unilateral defect in arousal (alerting) induced by a defect in a corticolimbic reticular loop. In general, the loop postulated is similar to that proposed by Sokolov (63). The cortex is responsible for stimulus analysis—i.e., novel versus nonnovel; biological significance versus nonsignificance. If a stimulus is novel or significant, corticofugal impulses direct the reticular system to activate the cortex.

For the proposed loop to be possible, there should be both corticofugal projections to the reticular system and reticular projections to the cortex. Unilateral lesions of the reticular formation or of another formation in the loop should produce neglect. In regard to the corticofugal input into the reticular system, Nauta (52) demonstrated that the cingulate gyrus has extensive connections with the mesencephalic reticular formation. Astruc (2) showed a connection between the dorsolateral frontal lobe (i.e., arcuate gyrus) and the mesencephalic reticular system. French, Hernandez-Peon, and Livingston (21) studied corticofugal pathways to the reticular system with evoked potentials and physiologic neurono-graphic techniques. These investigators found that corticofugal pathways arose from the arcuate gyrus (dorsolateral frontal lobe), cingulate gyrus, sensorimotor cortex, and posterior parietal and superior temporal gyrus regions. Segundo, Naguet, and Buser (61) were able to induce both diffuse electrocortical and behavioral arousal in the monkey by subconvulsive stimulation of the arcuate gyrus, the posterior parietal superior temporal regions, and the cingulate gyrus. The cortical sites for reticular firing and for behavioral and electroencephalo-graphic (EEG) arousal are identical to those areas that produce neglect when ablated.

Reeves and Hagamen (57) induced a neglect-like state in cats by mesencephalic lesions, and Watson and co-workers (73) effected neglect in monkeys by making discrete lesions in the mesencephalic reticular formation.

As regards the reticular fibers to the cortex, no direct connection has been demonstrated between the reticular formation and the cortex. The mesencephalic reticular formation appears to send fibers to the hypothalamic, preoptic, and septal areas. The rostral portion of the mesencephalon also sends fibers to the caudate and lentiform nuclei (12). There are also descending fibers that go to the thalamic nuclei (i.e., intralaminar and central median nucleus). Regarding corti-cal desynchronization, it appears that lesions in the mesencephalic reticular formation block EEG desynchronization even to thalamic stimulation (74).

Two ascending routes have been postulated. The dorsal route, via the thalamus, is important in recruitment phenomena; the ventral route is important for desynchronization (13). As previously mentioned, the lateral hypothalamus re-ceives fibers from the mesencephalic reticular formation (as does the substantia innominata). Recently, Kievit and Kuypers (41) have demonstrated that these basal forebrain areas project to the cortex; and Van Hoesen (68) has suggested that these areas may be an important relay in the ascending limb of a corticolim-bic reticular loop proposed by Heilman and Valenstein (31) and Watson and associates (72). Marshall, Turner, and Teitelbaum (49) ablated the lateral hypo-thalamus and produced neglect. Included in their lesion was the ascending reticu-lar hypothalamic pathway, as well as other pathways. Their findings give support to the concept that these basal forebrain areas may be important in the mediation of arousal. Kievit and Kuypers (41) also noted that the connections from the basal forebrain areas to the cortex are comparable in some respects with the ascending monoaminergic pathways, and they thought that the monoaminergic pathways connected with the basal forebrain projection system because their projection to the cortex traversed the lateral hypothalamus and substantia innominata. Unger-stedt (66) unilaterally removed the nigrostriatal system by stereotactic injections of 6-hydroxydopamine hydrobromide and produced the unilateral neglect syn-drome.

Lindsley and associates (46) made bilateral lesions of the midbrain tegmentum in cats. Electroencephalograms recorded from these animals showed bilateral slow waves. If neglect is a unilateral arousal defect, then one would expect unilateral EEG slowing in subjects with this syndrome. Berlucchi (8) and Reeves and Hagamen (57) demonstrated unilateral EEG slowing in cats. Watson and colleagues (73) extended these observations to monkeys. Animals with unilateral neglect from cortical lesions (frontal arcuate gyrus, cingulate gyrus) also demonstrated unilateral EEG slowing (69).

We (69) have also studied 23 patients with unilateral neglect and compared them with 20 subjects with aphasia without neglect. Twenty-two of the 23 patients with unilateral neglect demonstrated diffuse ipsilateral slowing. Seven of the 20 in the aphasic group showed ipsilateral slowing. The difference between these groups is significant. There were no significant differences between these groups in the frequency of positive brain scans, the size of the scans, or the day between onset of their ictus and the EEG recording. The lesions of most patients were in the parietal lobe (14 of 19 with positive scans). We are not certain why the one subject with unilateral neglect did not show diffuse slowing. Perhaps this patient represents a dissociation of the phasic and tonic arousal systems (62,63). If diffuse slowing is present, there is a loss of tonic and phasic arousal, and neglect will be present. However, neglect may also be present with a loss of phasic arousal, although tonic arousal is preserved. Unfortunately unilateral stimulation was not performed on this patient to ascertain whether there was desynchronization of his EEG.

Although the EEG data appear to support the arousal hypothesis of neglect, they do not rule out the possibility that asymmetrical sensory input is producing these EEG changes. Unlike the routine EEG, the evoked potential (EP) is a macropotential that is time-locked to a sensory stimulus and demonstrates several components. In general, the early components of the EP are thought to be an electrical representation of specific sensory conduction, whereas later components reflect arousal, alerting, and attentional neural activities. It would appear then that the EP would be well suited to separate the sensory from the attentional postulates. Watson and co-workers (70) studied three unanesthetized *Macaca speciosa* by electrically stimulating the peroneal nerve and recording EPs from the cortical hind limb area. Sixty-four nonpainful stimuli were applied to each leg. Preoperative recordings were taken for 7 days, and then the animals underwent an arcuate gyrus ablation that induced unilateral neglect. Postoperatively, recordings were then taken from the 3rd through 9th days. The amplitude and latency were measured for each of the major waves. Comparing the changes in these waves from the preoperative to the postoperative conditions between the lesioned and nonlesioned sides demonstrated no significant interaction for the early waves, but there was a significant interaction for the late waves (i.e., latency of N_2, P_3, and amplitude of P_3). These findings appear to detract from the sensory hypothesis and give support to the attention-arousal hypothesis.

Watson, Miller, and Heilman (71) also performed a behavioral experiment to help determine whether the defective orienting response seen in neglect is a result of an attention-arousal or of a sensory defect. Three monkeys were trained to open a left door in response to right-side stimulation and a right door to left-side stimulation. After training, each monkey received a unilateral lesion, either frontal arcuate or intralaminar nucleus, which induced severe neglect. No monkey would orient to unilateral stimuli. When the monkeys were touched on the side contralateral to the lesion (i.e., the neglected side), they opened the appropriate door ipsilateral to the lesions, which was the trained response; however, when they were stimulated on the normal side, they either failed to open any door, or opened the door ipsilateral to their lesion even though they had been trained to do the opposite.

In a similar fashion, we have examined four human patients with severe left-side unilateral neglect (33). These patients were instructed to raise their left hand to the right-side stimuli and their right hand to left-side stimulation. All four patients made more errors when the normal side (right) was stimulated than when the abnormal side was stimulated; they more frequently raised the right hand to the right-side stimulation than the left hand to left-side stimulation.

Although both the experimental animals and the human patients tended to have a paucity of movements on the neglected side, both experimental groups demonstrated enough strength to perform the task. In the animal experiments, the lesion never involved "motor areas." These experiments clearly demonstrate that the defective orienting response seen with the neglect syndrome cannot be explained by a sensory hypothesis. If the defect were a sensory one, then the animal would not have opened the door ipsilateral to the lesion when it was stimulated on the side contralateral to the lesion. This is clearly what our subjects did best.

Unlike other reaction patterns to sensory stimuli, the orienting reaction is preparatory rather than consummatory (47). Increased arousal not only reduces threshold to incoming stimuli but also prepares the organism for action. Lesions that induce the unilateral neglect syndrome produce a unilateral reduction of arousal, and, because one hemisphere is hypoaroused, it cannot prepare for action and therefore is akinetic.

Because animals and patients often have a paucity of movements contralateral to a hemispheric lesion, even though the lesion does not involve the traditional motor areas, this poverty of movement (hypokinesia) is being produced not by a motor defect, but rather by an attentional or arousal defect. Frequently, when a patient with severe neglect is asked to bisect a line, he quarters the line; when asked to draw a daisy, he will draw half a daisy. The abnormality is often explained as a sensory defect (homonymous hemianopia). Interestingly, patients who are blind, from peripheral disease, can still draw a daisy (i.e., one does not need vision to draw a simple object). We suggest that the reason the patients with neglect draw only half a daisy is that they have a unilateral akinesis. This unilateral akinesis is not limited to the extremities on one side of the body; it is an akinesis to any stimuli that come to the hypoaroused hemisphere.

INTERHEMISPHERIC HYPOTHESES

Most of the interhemispheric hypotheses have been invoked to explain extinction. Bender and Furlow (6,7) studied a patient and noted that the defect in sensation was increased by the phenomenon of rivalry and dominance from the intact hemisphere. Nathan (51) noted that, although a stimulus was perceived on the abnormal side, it would become imperceptible when a stimulus was applied to the normal side. Nathan therefore postulated that the normal side was suppressing the abnormal side. Reider (58) and Furmanski (22) also thought that the normal hemisphere suppressed the abnormal hemisphere. The basic mechanism underlying all these theories is suppression.

The concept of cortical suppressor action has long been abandoned (perhaps prematurely). Birch, Belmont, and Karp (9) proposed an interhemispheric mechanism that does not rely on a suppressor. These authors postulated that the damaged hemisphere processes information more slowly than the undamaged hemisphere does and, because it processes information more slowly, it is more subject to interference from the normal side. These authors supported their hypothesis by demonstrating that stimulation of the intact side before stimulation of the abnormal side induced extinction; however, when the abnormal side was stimulated first, extinction was reduced. The arousal hypothesis presented earlier cannot completely explain the extinction phenomenon, but defective arousal may be responsible for the slowed responses.

There is an alternative postulate to explain extinction (32). As previously mentioned, as an organism with neglect improves, it goes from the stage of unresponsivity and allesthesia (in which the organism always orients to its normal side) to the stage of extinction (in which it can orient to either side with unilateral stimulation). During the extinction stage, the ability to orient to the abnormal side may be mediated, at least in part, by the normal hemisphere. With simultaneous stimulation perhaps the normal hemisphere is preoccupied with the contralateral stimuli and, therefore, is unresponsive to the ipsilateral stimuli. Our theory is one of distraction rather than of suppression.

Kinsbourne (43) has also proposed a theory to explain the neglect phenomenon. He expressed the belief that each hemisphere inhibits the other by callosal mechanisms and that the syndrome of neglect is being produced by a decrease in transcallosal inhibitory influences on the normal hemisphere. Although an imbalance between the orientational tendencies would appear to explain the head and eye deviation seen in neglect, the same type of orientational imbalance could be explained by a decrease of activity (hypoarousal) of the lesioned hemisphere. As previously mentioned, there is little evidence to suggest a suppressor. Furthermore, callosal lesions do not prevent neglect (20), rather they appear to make it worse (67). Bilateral lesions in areas known to produce unilateral neglect do not improve behavior, but rather produce an akinetic mute state (31,72).

Many of our patients with the unilateral neglect syndrome have, as Battersby, Bender, and Pollack (3) suggested, an altered mental status. Although they have a lesion restricted to one hemisphere, they look like the akinetic mute with bilateral frontal or cingulate disease. We think these patients are hypokinetic because they have bilateral arousal (alerting) defects, the lesioned side being more hypoaroused than the nonlesioned side. If one subscribes to our attention-arousal hypothesis of neglect, there is some evidence to support the foregoing clinical observations. Regarding physiologic support, when Moruzzi and Magoun (50) unilaterally stimulated the reticular system, the animal demonstrated bilateral activation. The ipsilateral cortex, however, showed a stronger arousal response than did the contralateral cortex. When Segundo, Naguet, and Buser (61) showed that cortical stimulation could effect behavioral and EEG arousal, they found that unilateral stimulation induced bilateral arousal. The anatomy of reticulocortical projections has not been completely elucidated; however, Rossi and Brodal (59) studied corticoreticular pathways and demonstrated that each hemisphere projects bilaterally to the reticular formation.

There is also some behavioral evidence. Gainotti and Tiacci (24) and Albert (1) noted that, although patients with unilateral neglect make more errors on the side contralateral to their lesions, they also make more errors on the side ipsilateral to a lesion than do controls. Reaction times are evidence of arousal and correlate with EEG evidence of arousal (45). Recently, we have examined the visual reaction times of seven patients with unilateral neglect. Although the stimulus was delivered to both fields and the hand opposite the nonlesioned cortex performed the reaction times, our neglect patients' reaction times were very slow. A warning stimulus reduces reaction time because it increases arousal (45), but even when warning and reaction time stimuli were given to the side ipsilateral to the lesion, there was no significant reduction of reaction time (29). As another measure of arousal we also used a galvanic skin response. We recorded from the hand ipsilateral to the lesion, and we stimulated this same hand. With the galvanic skin response set at maximal sensitivity and with electrical stimuli that were judged by the patient as uncomfortable, there was no galvanic skin response or the response was minimal. Unlike our neglect patients, aphasic controls showed an excellent response (29).

Most of the hypokinetic patients we see with the unilateral neglect syndrome appear to have right-hemisphere lesions. Our clinical observations would suggest that neglect from right-hemisphere lesions produces a greater ipsilateral arousal (alerting) defect than do lesions of the left hemisphere. There appears to be some indirect evidence to support this observation.

DeRenzi and Faglioni (19) studied patients with unilateral lesions. In such patients, when the hand ipsilateral to the lesion was used, one would have expected normal reaction times; but these investigators found that reaction times were slowed from lesions in either hemisphere. They also found that lesions of the right hemisphere caused greater slowing than did lesions of the left hemisphere. To explain this phenomenon, DeRenzi and Faglioni suggested that reaction time is proportional to the extent and severity of a cerebral lesion without respect to its focus. They thought that, since right-hemisphere lesions tend to be less symptomatic than left-hemisphere lesions, their patients with right-hemisphere disease had bigger lesions. Subsequently, Howes and Boller (38) studied reaction times in brain-damaged subjects. They demonstrated that lesions of the left hemisphere tend to be larger than those of the right hemisphere; however, the patients with lesions on the right had greater slowing of their reaction times than did those with left-hemisphere lesions. In patients with cortical lesions, the greatest slowing appeared with posterior parietal lesions, the nondominant lesions producing the greatest defect. As previously mentioned, it has been demonstrated that simple reaction time correlates with EEG evidence of activation (45). It has also been observed that neglect is most often associated with nondominant parietal lesions (1,11,15,48). Although Howes and Boller (38) alluded to a loss of topographical sense as perhaps being responsible for their subjects' prolonged reaction times, they were careful not to draw any conclusions about why nondominant parietal lobe lesions produced slowed reaction times. We would propose that their data support our hypothesis and suggest that a unilateral nondominant parietal lesion with neglect produces a bilateral defect in arousal, the lesioned hemisphere being even less aroused than is the nonlesioned hemisphere. Unfortunately, Howes and Boller did not report testing their patients for neglect. However, of interest is that, of the neglect patients we previously mentioned with abnormal galvanic skin reaction and reaction times (to stimuli delivered to their normal side), all but one had right-hemisphere lesions. There are, however, additional data on normal subjects that also provide some evidence for a specific role of the right parietal region in attentional arousal. Beck, Dustman, and Sakai (4) noted that when the evoked potential was used as a measure of attention, the greatest amplitude change with increased attention was always seen in those responses recorded from the right parietal leads.

Recently, Bowers and Heilman (10) gave 16 normal subjects either a verbal or nonverbal warning stimulus followed by a neutral reaction-time stimulus. Reaction times by the right hand were significantly faster with verbal warning stimuli than with nonverbal warning stimuli. There were, however, no significant differences for the left hand between verbal and nonverbal warning stimuli. Wood and Goff (77) reported that auditory evoked potentials were different in the left hemisphere, although identical over the right during linguistic and nonlinguistic analyses of the same signal. Perhaps both Bowers and Heilman (10) and Wood and Goff (77) have demonstrated that the left hemisphere is alerted by a specific stimulus—language—whereas, the right hemisphere is alerted by all stimuli.

Moreover, if right-side lesions do induce a more severe hypokinesia than left-side lesions and if the mechanism underlying the hypokinesia is hypoarousal, it would appear that the right hemisphere has more of an influence on left-hemisphere arousal than vice versa.

Patients with neglect frequently appear inappropriately indifferent (18,23). Although all of Gainotti's patients had unilateral neglect, he did not think that the neglect syndrome was important in producing the flattened affect seen in these patients. It has been demonstrated that patients with right temporoparietal lesions and neglect have difficulty with tonal contour processing and cannot comprehend or express affective tones (28,65). Schachter (60) has postulated that emotional states are a function of physiologic arousal and a cognition appropriate to the state of arousal. Since patients with right temporoparietal lesions have both a defect in intonational contour processing and a bilateral (but asymmetrical) defect in phasic arousal, it follows that they would have a flattened affect and appear to be indifferent (25).

MECHANICS UNDERLYING HEMISPHERIC ASYMMETRIES OF NEGLECT

In a previous paper, we (32) reviewed some of the evidence that right-side lesions produce a more profound defect than do left-side lesions. We discussed four theories that have been postulated to explain this asymmetry: (a) Neglect is more severe with right-side lesions because the right side is also concerned with visuo-spatial processing (1,48). (b) It is possible that there are more excitatory neurotransmitters on the left side of the brain, producing a propensity to orient to the right. Right-side lesions would then produce a greater asymmetry of the orienting response than would lesions of the left side (32). (c) Perhaps the corticoreticular loop responsible for alerting (activation, phasic arousal) is more discretely organized in the right hemisphere than it is in the left hemisphere (32). If corticofugal fibers are more discretely organized on the right, a lesion of the cortex would effect not only a more severe defect of the orienting response to contralesional stimuli, because of decreased ipsilateral input into the reticular system, but also a greater bilateral arousal defect because a cortical lesion would also interfere with input into the contralateral side of the reticular system. (d) Since patients think in words and verbally communicate with their physician, language produces left-hemisphere activation (10,42,44). Left-hemisphere activation would minimize an imbalance from left-hemisphere lesions and enhance an imbalance caused by right-hemisphere lesions (43).

Currently there is no anatomic or physiologic evidence to support the second and third theories. In response to the last theory, we recently (26) examined six patients with unilateral neglect from right-side lesions. All the subjects were presented with six trials of crossing-out tasks similar to the one used by Albert (1). In three of the crossing-out tasks the subjects were presented with sheets containing three six-letter words (i.e., school, center, doctor) distributed across a card. The subjects were instructed to cross out one of the words (e.g., doctor) wherever they saw it on the card. In the three other crossing-out tasks the patients were presented with a card that had lines oriented in one of three directions (vertical, horizontal, or diagonal). Again, the subjects were instructed to cross out only a specific type of line (e.g., vertical) wherever they saw it on the card. The lines were the same size as the words, and there were just as many lines as words on each card. All six subjects with left-side neglect demonstrated less neglect—crossed out more lines and went further to their left on the page—in the visuospatial condition than they did in the language condition. These results give partial support to Kinsbourne's hypothesis, but we are not certain that the mild effect seen in our study can account for the gross asymmetries seen with the neglect syndrome. To ascertain how important asymmetrical cognitive processing is in the production of hemispheric asymmetries of neglect, Albert's (1) study must be repeated using our paradigm.

OTHER BEHAVIORAL CHANGES ASSOCIATED WITH THE NEGLECT SYNDROME

Our discussion of the unilateral neglect syndrome has dealt with the defects of the orienting responses seen with these patients. Patients with neglect can also demonstrate: (a) denial of illness (75), (b) memory defects (34), (c) motor impersistence (39), or (d) visuospatial defects (48). A discussion of all the above is beyond the scope of this chapter. It would appear, however, that a defect in the orienting response may be implicated in some of the foregoing defects. Because the lesions that produce neglect in man are frequently cortical, many of the above defects may be cortical processing defects, which accompany the disorder of the orienting response but have a different mechanism. The importance of defective orienting and arousal in the production of the above defects will have to be elucidated by further research.

REFERENCES

1. Albert, M. C. (1973): A simple test of visual neglect. *Neurology,* 23:658–664.
2. Astruc, J. (1971): Corticofugal connections of area 8 (frontal eye field) in *Macaca mulatta. Brain Res.,* 33:241–256.
3. Battersby, W. S., Bender, M. B., and Pollack, M. (1956): Unilateral spatial agnosia (inattention) in patients with cerebral lesions. *Brain,* 79:68–93.
4. Beck, E. C., Dustman, R. E., and Sakai, M. (1969): Electrophysiological correlates of selective attention. In: *Attention in Neurophysiology,* edited by C. R. Evans and R. B. Mulholland, p. 412. Appleton Century Crofts, New York.
5. Bender, M. B. (1952): *Disorders in Perception.* Charles C Thomas, Springfield, Ill.
6. Bender, M. B., and Furlow, C. T. (1944): Phenomenon of visual extinction and binocular rivalry mechanism. *Trans. Am. Neurol. Assoc.,* 70:87–93.
7. Bender, M. B., and Furlow, C. T. (1945): Phenomenon of visual extinction in homonymous fields and psychological principles involved. *Arch. Neurol. Psychiatry,* 53:29–33.
8. Berlucchi, G. (1966): Electroencephalographic studies in split brain cats. *Electroencephalogr. Clin. Neurophysiol.,* 20:348–356.
9. Birch, H. G., Belmont, I., and Karp, E. (1967): Delayed information processing and extinction following cerebral damage. *Brain,* 90:113–130.
10. Bowers, D., and Heilman, K. M. (1976): Material specific hemispheric arousal. *Neuropsychologia,* 14:123–127.
11. Brain, W. R. (1941): Visual disorientation with special reference to lesions of the right cerebral hemisphere. *Brain,* 64:244–272.
12. Brodal, A. (1956): *The Reticular Formation of the Brainstem.* Charles C Thomas, Springfield, Ill.
13. Brodal, A. (1969): *Neurological Anatomy,* pp. 334–335. Oxford University Press, London.
14. Critchley, M. (1949): Tactile inattention with reference to partietal lesions. *Brain,* 72:538–561.
15. Critchley, M. (1966): *The Parietal Lobes.* Hafner, New York.
16. Davis, B., and Benevento, L. A. (1975): Single cell responses to auditory and visual stimuli in the preoccipital gyrus and superior temporal gyrus in the macaque monkey. Presented at the Society of Neuroscience, New York.
17. Denny-Brown, D., and Banker, B. Q. (1954): Amorphosynthesis from left parietal lesions. *Arch. Neurol. Psychiatry,* 71:302–313.

18. Denny-Brown, D., Meyer, J. S., and Horenstein, S. (1952): The significance of perceptual rivalry resulting from parietal lesion. *Brain,* 75:434–471.
19. DeRenzi, E., and Faglioni, P. (1965): The comparative efficiency of intelligence and vigilance tests detecting hemispheric damage. *Cortex,* 1:410–433.
20. Eidelberg, E., and Schwartz, A. J. (1971): Experimental analysis of the extinction phenomenon in monkeys. *Brain,* 94:91–108.
21. French, J. D., Hernandez-Peon, R., and Livingston, R. (1955): Projections from the cortex to cephalic brainstem (reticular formation) in monkeys. *J. Neurophysiol.,* 18:74–95.
22. Furmanski, A. R. (1950): The phenomena of sensory suppression. *Arch. Neurol. Psychiatry,* 63:205–217.
23. Gainotti, G. (1972): Emotional behavior and hemispheric side of the lesion. *Cortex,* 8:41–55.
24. Gainotti, G., and Tiacci, C. (1971): The relationships between disorders of visual perception and unilateral spatial neglect. *Neuropsychologia,* 9:451–458.
25. Heilman, K. M. (1976): Affective disorders associated with right-hemisphere disease. Presented at The Academy of Aphasia, Oct 11, 1976, Miami, Florida.
26. Heilman, K. M., and Watson, R. T. (1977): Changes in the symptoms of neglect induced by changing task strategy. (*In preparation.*)
27. Heilman, K. M., Pandya, D. M., Karol, E. A., and Geschwind, N. (1971): Auditory inattention. *Arch. Neurol.,* 24:323–325.
28. Heilman, K. M., Scholes, R., and Watson, R. T. (1975): Auditory affective agnosia: Disturbed comprehension of affective speech. *J. Neurol. Neurosurg. Psychiatry,* 38:69–72.
29. Heilman, K. M., Schwartz, H., and Watson, R. (1977): The galvanic skin response in patients with abnormal emotional reaction from brain dysfunction. *Neurology,* 27:350.
30. Heilman, K. M., and Valenstein, E. (1972): Auditory neglect in man. *Arch. Neurol.,* 26:32–35.
31. Heilman, K. M., and Valenstein, E. (1972): Frontal lobe neglect in man. *Neurology,* 22:660–664.
32. Heilman, K. M., and Watson, R. T. (1977): The neglect syndrome—A unilateral defect of the orienting response. In: *Lateralization in the Nervous System,* edited by S. Harnad. Academic Press, New York.
33. Heilman, K. M., and Watson, R. T. Unilateral akinesia associated with the neglect syndrome. (*In preparation.*)
34. Heilman, K. M., Watson, R. T., and Schulman, H. (1974): A unilateral memory defect. *J. Neurol. Neurosurg. Psychiatry,* 37:790–793.
35. Holmes, G. (1918): Disturbances of vision by cerebral lesions. *Br. J. Ophthalmol.,* 2:353–384.
36. Holmes, G. (1919): Disturbances of visual space perception. *Br. Med. J.,* 2:230–233.
37. Holmes, G., and Horrax, G. (1919): Disturbances of spatial orientation and visual attention with loss of stereoscopic vision. *Arch. Neurol. Psychiatry,* 1:385–407.
38. Howes, D., and Boller, F. (1975): Simple reaction time: Evidence for focal impairment from lesions of the right hemisphere. *Brain,* 98:317–332.
39. Joynt, R. J., Benton, A. L., and Fogel, M. L. (1962): Behavioral and pathological correlates of motor impersistence. *Neurology,* 12:876–881.
40. Kennard, M. A., and Ectors, L. (1938): Forced circling movements in monkeys following lesions of the frontal lobes. *J. Neurophysiol.,* 1:45–54.
41. Kievit, J., and Kuypers, H. G. J. M. (1975): Basal forebrain and hypothalamic connections to frontal and parietal cortex in rhesus monkeys. *Science,* 187:660–662.
42. Kinsbourne, M. (1970): The cerebral basis of lateral asymmetries in attention. *Acta Psychol.,* 33:193–201.
43. Kinsbourne, M. (1970): A model for the mechanism of unilateral neglect of space. *Trans. Am. Neurol. Assoc.,* 95:143.
44. Kinsbourne, M. (1974): Direction of gaze and distribution of cerebral thought processes. *Neuropsychologia,* 12:270–281.
45. Lansing, R. W., Schwartz, E., and Lindsley, D. B. (1959): Reaction time and EEG activation under alerted and nonalerted conditions. *J. Exp. Psychol.,* 58:1–7.
46. Lindsley, D. B., Schreiner, L. J., Knowles, W. B., and Magoun, H. W. (1950): Behavioral and EEG changes following chronic brainstem lesions in cat. *Electroencephalogr. Clin. Neurophysiol.,* 2:483–498.
47. Lynn, R. (1966): *Attention, Arousal and the Orientation Reaction.* Pergamon Press, Oxford.
48. McFie, J., Piercy, M. F., and Zangwill, O. L. (1950): Visual spatial agnosia associated with lesions of the right hemisphere. *Brain,* 73:167–190.

49. Marshall, J. F., Turner, B. H., and Teitelbaum, P. (1971): Sensory neglect produced by lateral hypothalamic damage. *Science,* 174:523–525.
50. Moruzzi, G., and Magoun, H. W. (1949): Brainstem reticular formation and activation of the EEG. *Electroencephalogr. Clin. Neurophysiol.,* 1:455–473.
51. Nathan, P. W. (1946): On simultaneous bilateral stimulation of the body in a lesion of the parietal lobe. *Brain,* 69:325–334.
52. Nauta, W. J. H. (1964): Some efferent connections of the prefrontal cortex in the monkey. In: *The Frontal Granular Cortex and Behavior,* edited by J. M. Warren and K. Akert. McGraw-Hill, New York.
53. Obersteiner, H. (1881): On allochiria—a peculiar sensory disorder. *Brain,* 4:153–163.
54. Pandya, D. M., and Kuypers, H. G. J. M. (1969): Cortico-cortical connections in the rhesus monkey. *Brain Res.,* 13:13–36.
55. Paterson, A., and Zangwill, O. L. (1944): Disorders of visual space perception associated with lesions of the right cerebral hemisphere. *Brain,* 67:331–358.
56. Poppelreuter, W. L. (1917): *Die psychischen Schädigungen durch Kopfschuss im Krieg 1914–1916: Die Störungen der niederen und höheren Leistungen durch Verletzungen des Oksipitalhirns. Vol. 1.* Leopold Voss, Leipzig. [Referred to by Critchley, M. (1949): *Brain,* 72:540.]
57. Reeves, A. G., and Hagamen, W. D. (1971): Behavioral and EEG asymmetry following unilateral lesions of the forebrain and midbrain of cats. *Electroencephalogr. Clin. Neurophysiol.,* 30:83–86.
58. Reider, N. (1946): Phenomena of sensory suppression. *Arch. Neurol. Psychiatry,* 55:583–590.
59. Rossi, G. F., and Brodal, A. (1956): Corticofugal fibers to the brainstem reticular formation. An experimental study in the cat. *J. Anat.,* 90:42–63.
60. Schachter, S. (1975): Cognition and peripheralist centralist controversies in motivation and emotion. In: *The Handbook of Psychobiology,* edited by M. S. Gazzaniga and C. Blakemore, pp. 529–564. Academic Press, New York.
61. Segundo, J. P., Naguet, R., and Buser, P. (1955): Effects of cortical stimulation on electrocortical activity in monkeys. *J. Neurophysiol.,* 18:236–245.
62. Sharpless, S. K., and Jasper, H. H. (1956): Habituation of the arousal reaction. *Brain,* 79:655–669.
63. Sokolov, Y. N. (1963): *Perception and the Conditioned Reflex.* Pergamon Press, Oxford.
64. Sprague, J. M., Chambers, W. W., and Stellar, E. (1961): Attentive, affective and adaptive behavior in the cat. *Science,* 133:165–173.
65. Tucker, D., Watson, R. T., and Heilman, K. M. (1976): Affective discrimination and evocation in patients with right parietal disease. *Neurology,* 26:354.
66. Ungerstedt, U. (1973): Selective lesions of central catecholamine pathways: Application in functional studies. In: *Neuroscience Research, Vol. 5, Chemical approaches to brain function,* edited by S. Ehrenpreis and I. Kopin, pp. 73–96. Academic Press, New York.
67. Valenstein, E., Pandya, D. M., and Heilman, K. M. (*Unpublished observations.*)
68. Van Hoesen, G. (1976): (*Personal communication.*)
69. Watson, R. T., and Heilman, K. M. (1977): The electroencephalogram in neglect. (*In preparation.*)
70. Watson, R. T., Miller, B. D., and Heilman, K. M. (1977): Evoked potential in neglect. Arch. Neurol., 34:224–227.
71. Watson, R. T., Miller, B. D., and Heilman, K. M. (1977): (*In preparation.*)
72. Watson, R. T., Heilman, K. M., Cauthen, J. C., and King, F. A. (1973): Nonsensory neglect after cingulectomy. *Neurology,* 23:1003–1007.
73. Watson, R. T., Heilman K. M., Miller, B. D., and King, F. A. (1974): Neglect after mesencephalic reticular formation lesions. *Neurology,* 24:294–298.
74. Weinburger, N. M., Velasco, M., and Lindsley, D. B. (1965): Effect of lesions upon thalamically induced electrocortical desynchronization and recruiting. *Electroencephalogr. Clin. Neurophysiol.,* 18:369–377.
75. Weinstein, E. A., and Kahn, R. L. (1955): *Denial of Illness.* Charles C Thomas, Springfield, Ill.
76. Welch, K., and Stuteville, P. (1958): Experimental production of neglect in monkeys. *Brain,* 81:341–347.
77. Wood, C., and Goff, W. (1971): Auditory evoked potentials during speech perception. *Science,* 173:1248–1251.
78. Yin, T. C. T., Lynch, J. C., Talbot, W. H., and Mountcastle, V. B. (1975): Neuronal mechanisms of the parietal lobe for directed visual attentions. Presented at the Society of Neuroscience, New York.

DISCUSSION

Dr. Friedland: What is the evidence you have that extinction can be considered a manifestation of hemi-inattention by itself?

Dr. Heilman: This explanation is hypothetical. When the contralateral side is stimulated, sensory information is transmitted not only to the contralateral hemisphere but also to the ipsilateral hemisphere. Thus, allesthesia need not be caused by a perceptual error of the impaired hemisphere, but perhaps by the normal hemisphere responding as if the stimulus were a signal for it to perform. This hypothesis would imply some type of reciprocal interhemispheric inhibition (e.g., under normal circumstances the hemisphere contralateral to a stimulus may inhibit the ipsilateral hemisphere from performing). During recovery the organism usually goes from the stage of allesthesia to extinction. At this stage the normal hemisphere can direct an appropriate response to either a contralateral or ipsilateral stimulus. However, when simultaneous stimuli are presented, the contralateral stimulus predominates (i.e., the normal hemisphere is doing its own thing).

Dr. Cohn: Your theoretical structure about the two sides of the brain, one of it doing its own thing, I think that's what Dr. Joynt was showing in his evoked response. You saw that with the single response on the, say, median nerve, you got a lower amplitude on the ipsilateral side. That's all. And, therefore, what I think is happening is what you are saying and it's not theoretical. You have a real conditioned inhibition of the ipsilateral response and you learn not to use it. Under the conditions in which something breaks down, this becomes a determinant of phenomena. I think that's very clear. Period.

Dr. Heilman: I agree.

Dr. Friedland: What is the evidence for believing that the corticoreticular loop is more discretely organized in the right hemisphere?

Dr. Heilman: This is hypothetical. We have no direct evidence, as I have indicated.

Advances in Neurology, Vol. 18, edited by E. A.
Weinstein and R. P. Friedland. Raven Press,
New York © 1977.

Extinction and Other Patterns of Sensory Interaction

Morris B. Bender

Department of Neurology, Mount Sinai Medical School, New York, New York 10029

I would like to begin by discussing a phenomenon that goes back to Hippocrates, who said that when you stimulate one area of the body you inhibit another. (A good example of this is the pickpocket who knows well that when a person is bumped on one side he will probably not feel his pocket being picked on the other.) This fact was rediscovered neurologically in the latter half of the nineteenth century, as is discussed by Friedland and Weinstein *(this volume).* If a person has a lesion on one side of the brain, for example the right, during bilateral simultaneous stimulations, the stimulus to the side opposite the lesion, namely the left, will not be perceived, even though, when tested separately with individual stimuli, the person responds correctly. This was first described by Oppenheim in 1885 (7). This interaction occurs across the vertical axis or the midline. Thus, if a person sees a light stimulus in his left field of vision and another stimulus is introduced into his right field of vision, he no longer sees the one on the left. This is an example of extinction across the vertical meridian (5). Extinction can occur across the horizontal plane, for example, in a situation in which the left superior quadrant of the visual field is affected and the inferior quadrant is relatively normal. If simultaneous stimuli are then introduced to both lower and superior quadrants, the stimulus delivered to the superior quadrant will disappear. I cite this to illustrate that the phenomenon of extinction does not necessarily involve an action only across the corpus callosum. It can occur on one side of the brain. These interactions across the midvertical on right and left side or on one side are illustrated by the following: In our face-hand test, interaction may occur either across the vertical or across the horizontal plane. If the face and hand are stimulated separately, each stimulus will be perceived correctly by the normal adult and older child. In patients with organic brain disease or senescence, and young, normal children below age 6 years, only the touch to the face will be appreciated. This interaction occurs across the midline when the left face and right hand are touched simultaneously. However, extinction also occurs in the hand when the right face and right hand are stimulated. Mistakes are more apt to occur if there is a certain asymmetry, but the face invariably is "dominant" over the hand. This is especially prominent in patients with organic mental syndrome, so that even with noxious pin prick stimuli, enough to draw blood, the patient insists he feels the pin only in his face. These same patients show no interaction when both hands are stimulated simultaneously. They do not make mistakes when two symmetrical right and left homologous skin areas are stimulated. Another effect of interaction is displacement. In the face-hand test, the hand percept may be "displaced" to the face (1). When touched, for instance on the right face and left hand, the patient indicates both cheeks when asked where he is touched. Also, in cases of severe diffuse organic brain disease, exosomesthesia is found. Here the patient, when touched simultaneously on the face and hand, localizes the face stimulus correctly but points out into space to indicate where he thinks he has perceived the hand stimulus. Exosomesthesia is commonly found in children up to the age of 6 years and in the elderly. The foregoing are examples of interactions that involve extrapersonal sensory space. The subject has a sensation of stimuli originating from outer space.

Bender and Diamond (3) have written about cross-modal or heteromodal interactions. For example, a tactile stimulus can be extinguished by a visual stimulus. When I examine an aged person or one with a severe organic mental syndrome, I touch my own face and the patient's hand, and while the patient is looking at me I ask him, "Where did I touch you?" He answers, "On my face" and touches his face. He extinguishes or does not perceive the tactile stimulus on the hand. Applying a visual stimulus, such as the waving of my hand in front of him, he may not feel the hand stimulus. If I touch only his hand, he will report it correctly. Moreover, a sound stimulus will also cause extinction of a single tactile stimulus. If I address the patient in a loud voice or intimidate him, he will not perceive the hand stimulus. Thus, there are interactions between visual, somatosensory, auditory stimuli, and, probably, "emotional" states. An auditory stimulus influences response in the somatosensory sphere and somatosensory stimulation can interfere with a visual or auditory response (2).

In cases of hemi-inattention, the patient does not seem to perceive any kind of stimulus applied to one side of the body. I consider the patient's whole perceptual world as a sphere, rather than a two-dimensional space. In a patient with a large right cerebral lesion, the left half of the perceptual sphere is defective, whereas the right half space is preserved but distorted. The new perceptual sphere in the patient with a right cerebral lesion is located completely to the right half of the midaxis. All modalities in the right-left sensory sphere surrounding the patient are governed by the remaining or "good" left cerebrum. I have never seen a patient with unilateral spatial hemi-inattention who had a disturbance only in vision; these patients have disturbances also in the somatosensory and auditory modalities. Some patients who have no demonstrable hearing defect can not localize sound on one side. In hemi-inattention there is a combination of defective percepts on one side, but there is also invariably impaired mental function. I've never seen a patient with hemi-inattention who had a normal mental status.

What happens when patients have bilateral involvement of the cerebral hemispheres? Do they have bilateral inattention? From previous observations the answer is yes. This may be found in patients with bilateral encephalopathy who may show bilateral constriction of the fields of vision (6). There was no gross impairment of vision during single target stimulation, but, when the patient was instructed to fixate a central point, the peripheral target was not seen. This was bilateral with resultant constriction of the field of vision, an example of inattention of peripheral vision (4). The converse of this is the theory of central dominance. Patients with bilateral encephalopathy may report small patterns in a visual display but neglect the larger patterns in which they are embedded (3). For example, they may see a series of number 3s that configured into a large 5. They can see the small 3s but not the large 5, even if outlined. These patients may also disregard moving objects in the peripheral fields of vision. There is interaction between central and peripheral visual fields, with resultant imperception in the periphery.

I am using the term imperception—although not quite in the same way as Hughlings Jackson did—to describe what has been called "unilateral hemi-inattention," "hemi-neglect," and "unilateral visuospatial agnosia" in a large contralateral cerebral lesion. The behavior involves extinction and its spatial variants, even allesthesia and changes in adaptation time. In the patient with diffuse cerebral dysfunction manifested by mental confusion, altered states of mental alertness make these phenomena more marked and widespread. In a patient with a unilateral morphological lesion and without mental changes, the intravenous injection of sodium amytal may produce a lateralized deficit with contralateral hemi-inattention, although there was no evidence of this prior to the injection. When a patient with a unilateral spatial deficit is required to perform tasks, such as reading, writing, and drawing, there are multiple sensory inputs, as well as motor output, with resultant interactions. Stimuli arising from the normal side interact with those arising from the affected side with resultant extinction of the defective stimuli. All inputs from right and left are directed or pulled to the intact sensory field. In such a situation, the head and eye movements are also integrally involved so that the subject looks and "pulls" to the "good" side. One can not attribute hemi-inattention solely to a lesion of one hemisphere or to the loss of some hypothetical function residing in that hemisphere. There is activity in the rest of the brain. A constant interaction is going on and, even after corpus callosum section, the interaction continues, mediated through structures on lower levels, e.g., the diencephalon and brainstem. The behavior of the organism is altered by a localized structural lesion, but the pattern and the degree of abnormality vary with the state of the remaining total cerebral function, including the degree of alertness. There may be unilateral imperception or inattention in a patient with unilateral lesion with mental dysfunction, but the same patient, when mentally clear, shows no inattention or imperception—only unilateral conventional sensory deficits.

REFERENCES

1. Bender, M. B. (1952): *Disorders in Perception (With Particular Reference to the Phenomena of Extinction and Displacement)*, pp. 1–109. Charles C Thomas, Springfield, Ill.

2. Bender, M. B. (1970): Perceptual interactions. In: *Modern Trends in Neurology,* edited by D. Williams, pp. 1–28. Butterworth, London.
3. Bender, M. B., and Diamond, S. P. (1970): Disorders in perception of space due to lesions of the nervous system. In: *Perception and Its Disorders. Res. Publ. Assoc. Res. Nerv. Ment. Dis.,* 48: 176–185.
4. Bender, M. B., and Diamond, S. P. (1975): Sensory interaction effects and their relation to the organization of perceptual space. In: *The Nervous System. Vol. 3: Human Communication and Its Disorders,* edited by D. B. Tower. Raven Press, New York.
5. Bender, M. B., and Furlow, L. T. (1945): Phenomenon of visual extinction in homonymous half fields and the psychologic principles involved. *Arch. Neurol. Psychiatry,* 53:29–33.
6. Goldstein, K. (1939): *The Organism.* American Book Co., New York.
7. Oppenheim, H. (1885): Ueber eine durch eine klinisch bisher nicht verwertete Untersuchungs-methode ermittelte Form der Sensibilitatsstorung bei einseitigen Erkrankungen des Grosshirns (Kurze Mitteilung). *Neurol. Centrabl.,* 23:529–533.

Advances in Neurology, Vol. 18, edited by E. A. Weinstein and R. P. Friedland. Raven Press, New York © 1977.

Symbol Retrieval Time as an Index of Attention

Robert Cohn

Department of Neurology, Howard University College of Medicine, Washington, D.C. 20059

Perceptual rivalry is of normal occurrence in all organismal input systems. Hemi-inattention is an elementary expression of perceptual rivalry which becomes manifest under conditions of disturbed brain function. To give some precision to these phenomena, I have carried out physiological experiments in man using summated cortical evoked responses. In one such physiological study (1), components of the rostral-caudal interaction were investigated. It was determined that stimuli presented within 25 msec of synchrony through the sciatic and median nerves usually had an interaction in which one pattern of the single nerve stimulation was either overwhelmed or an effectively new pattern of summated cortical response resulted. The proportion of hand and leg dominance as observed clinically was grossly recapitulated. In another study (2), homologous displacement resulting from simultaneously applied inhomogeneous paired stimuli could best be explained by a process of dissolution of normal conditioned inhibition.

In all this work, a basic assumption was that a strong interaction existed between the two cerebral hemispheres, most probably and most efficiently via the corpus callosum. The corpus callosum as an interhemispheric connector has been under investigation by behavioral, anatomical, and physiological brain scientists for a long time. In 1912 Poffenberger (7), using classical reaction time studies, determined in two subjects that the reaction times were between 5 and 6 msec longer when the sensory message had to be transmitted across the brain. In 1963 Efron (4), with an ingenious set of assumptions and measurements, determined that the interhemispheric transfer time was approximately 2 to 6 msec and that these data were processed by the hemisphere for speech.

Effectively these measurements were based on a scheme such as that shown in Fig. 1. In this diagram, the patterned input signal is conducted to the visual (or somesthetic) system of the right brain, and the left speech apparatus must be activated for utterance. Using a somewhat similar approach, I attempted a direct measurement of the transcallosal transit time by the method shown in Fig. 2. Two light cells were separated 21 inches apart on an optical bench. Numerals from 0 to 9, each 2 by 1¼ inches, were randomly applied in either visual field. The numbers were translucent white on a black background; the lamps were powered by tungsten filaments. The subject was placed approximately 1 ft in front

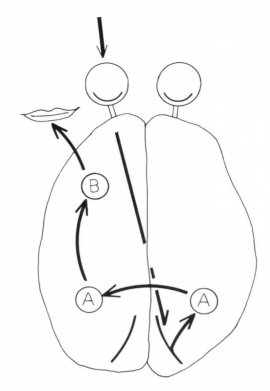

FIG. 1. Scheme of transcallosal processes in speech.

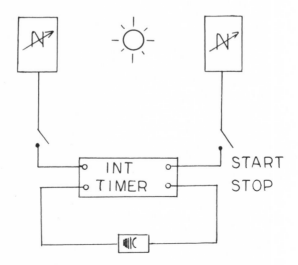

FIG. 2. Diagram of symbol processing method.

of the central position of the two cells; the head rested against a high-backed wooden chair. No attempt was made to fix the head. A red lamp was centered on the optical bench and was flashed for approximately 100 msec prior to the numeric light presentation. Random variable delays were made between each red light and numeric flash. The numeric flash presentations were of the order 100 to 200 msec. The switch that triggered the numeric signal triggered a Tektronix interval timer. The interval timer counting was terminated by the *initial* rise time of the output of a throat microphone operating into a Grayson-Stadler voice-operated relay. The attack time of this instrument was 20 msec by physical measurements. The subject was instructed to name the number presented as rapidly as possible. It seemed of some import that of the hundreds of numeric presentations, less than 2% were incorrectly named. The control subjects consisted of medical students and voluntary administrative personnel. Between 20 and 30 light presentations were made for each subject. It was interesting that no subject became significantly more precise with prolonged repeated presentations and that no greater coherence occurred around a fixed value of response with continued presentations. It was because of this fact that the presentations were confined to the number stated.

The results of such measurements are summarized in Table 1. These are the average response times of the normal subjects when randomly presented with numbers in the right and left visual fields. The extreme values were 407 and 596 msec for the numbers presented to the right field, and 336 and 611 msec for the left field. The mean value for the right field was 499 msec and, for the left, 491 msec; with standard deviations of 54.22 and 67.79, respectively. As noted above, with training and with increased presentations, no greater coherence was obtained. From the scatter, it became obvious that such data were not able to

TABLE 1. *Symbol naming times*

Controls	
Average	Responses
Right	Left
515.97	480.18
502.70	504.28
537.20	551.20
575.29	611.07
438.05	454.13
524.88	527.97
596.07	531.03
479.77	472.64
480.48	514.50
462.07	474.15
474.94	439.17
407.94	336.02

$\bar{X} = 499.61$; $\bar{X} = 491.39$; S.D. $= 54.22$;
S.D. $= 67.79$.

establish a consistent difference in transit times across the corpus callosum (or other cerebral interconnecting systems). Such measurements, however, could be used to demonstrate visual hemi-inattention in a reasonably precise way.

For example a patient presented with a left hemiparesis, including the face, mild pin prick changes over the left side, and visual hemi-inattention in the left homonymous fields as the result of a cerebral vascular occlusion of the right middle cerebral artery. The visual inattention was best demonstrated by the use of bilateral simultaneously applied stimuli. His graphic productions are shown in Fig. 3; the line on the left indicates the edge of the paper. It will be noted that there is an error in "ordering" in arithmetic; it is also observed that all cities are placed in the East Coast of the United States map. The "daisy" and "clockface" are not greatly distorted. The picture of a person was reasonably detailed and symmetric with multilinear contours. When the light stimuli were presented for a duration of less than 200 msec, the patient repeatedly failed to recognize the number in the left field of vision. When the numbers were allowed to remain on for ½ to 1 sec, he would almost invariably name the proper number. There were no evident eyeball movements, but electrodes were not placed around the orbits to make unequivocal measurements. In Fig. 4 it will be observed that the numbers applied to the right field were produced in approximately half the time required for the left field responses. It will be noted also that the right responses (normal side) at times were of much lower value than those of the control average of approximately 500 msec. This resulted from the patient's inability to completely direct the eyeballs to forward gaze. In the dark ambience, there was the tendency to direct the eyeballs to the seeing field. In individuals with dense homonymous hemianopia, it was remarkable that in the subdued light they continually rotated

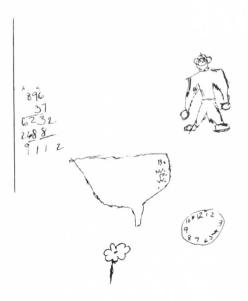

FIG. 3. Graphic productions of patient with hemi-inattention (visual).

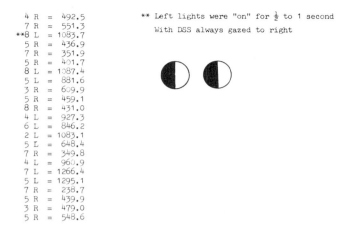

```
 4 R  =   492.5
 7 R  =   551.3
**8 L  =  1083.7
 5 R  =   436.9
 7 R  =   351.9
 5 R  =   401.7
 8 L  =  1087.4
 5 L  =   881.6
 3 R  =   609.9
 5 R  =   459.1
 8 R  =   431.0
 4 L  =   927.3
 6 L  =   846.2
 2 L  =  1083.1
 5 L  =   648.4
 7 R  =   349.8
 4 L  =   960.9
 7 L  =  1266.4
 5 L  =  1295.1
 7 R  =   238.7
 5 R  =   439.9
 3 R  =   479.0
 5 R  =   548.6
```

** Left lights were "on" for $\frac{1}{2}$ to 1 second

With DSS always gazed to right

FIG. 4. Symbol naming time in hemi-inattention patient.

their head toward the involved side so that it was quite impossible to even apply the stimuli into the unseeing field.

Although the transcallosal time measurement eluded this technique, it was believed that by changing the conditions of response, measurements could be obtained that might be related to symbol processing times. This was accomplished by having the same subjects signal phonetically when they recognized the light from either field, as *only the light,* without regard to the specific symbol recognition. Under these latter conditions, Table 2 showed an average response time of 316 msec. When this time was subtracted from the average time of relating to memory, retrieval, and naming (the symbol recognition time) this generated a

TABLE 2. *Average response to light (normals)*

Average	Controls	Responses
	369.67	
	363.12	
	367.88	
	237.96	
	328.36	
	386.27	
	324.21	
	305.09	
	366.54	
	280.13	
	258.84	
	209.71	

$\overline{X} = 316.48$; S.D. $= 58.54$.

TABLE 3. *Symbol processing times*

Controls	Patients
120.81	238.00
146.61	253.35
225.30	302.74
210.00	312.20
185.65	300.34
177.28	264.59
152.00	260.53
192.40	373.10
187.98	194.99[a]
162.27	269.96
	230.88
	274.47

$\bar{X} = 177.55$; $\bar{X} = 272.93$; S.D. = 32.70;
S.D. = 45.52; $T_S - T_L = T_{PT}$; PT = processing time.
[a] Cord lesion.

value that has been designated as the *symbol processing time*. The average value in the controls, first column of Table 3, was 177 msec. In patients with varying disorders such as peripheral neuropathy secondary to alcohol intoxication, hypothyroidism, liver disease, renal failure, and other metabolic disorders the average symbol processing time was approximately 277 msec, as shown in column two of Table 3. Such results were not unexpected from the clinical problems, but these results did give a measurable index of the intensity of the disturbed interaction potential of these people.

Another series of measurements were made, again using the visual apparatus as the input element for response. This system is shown in Fig. 5. The light signal was a single number repetitively applied in an irregular serial way from 100 to 400 times. The single number usually used was 2, 6, or 7 because of the rapid rise time of the wave front. The throat microphone output was simultaneously summated along with the summated cortical potentials derived from electrodes placed over the orthogonal projection of Broca's area. This area was localized

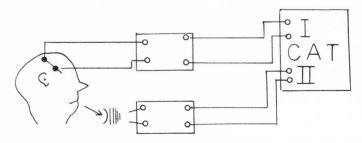

FIG. 5. Diagram of summated cortical evoked responses and microphone summations.

by first establishing the position of the rolandic fissure; this was obtained by a line drawn at an angle of 67° to the midsagittal plane, midway between the nasion and inion. The electrodes were placed 2 cm in front of this rolandic line, with the inferior electrode 8 cm distant from the midsagittal plane, and the superior electrode on the same line separated by 5 cm. The summated potentials of the evoked responses triggered by the visual stimuli were obtained with a CAT 1,000. The amplifiers were essentially flat between 1 and 3,000 Hz; the time constant was 0.4 sec. All records were in digital form as photographed from the face of the cathode ray tube of the CAT.

Figure 6 was obtained under these conditions. The upper line represents the summated cortical activity; the lower line, the summated microphone output. It should be recalled that only the rise time of the microphone response was utilized in the earlier measurements. From this figure, it will be observed that the first inflection leading into the positive going peak of cortical summated potential occurred at approximately 85 msec, with the positive maximum peak at 150 msec. It should be noted that the first inflection precedes the initial microphone deflection by at least 170 msec. That the initial deflection of the microphone summation is approximately 300 msec following the light flash confirms the earlier measurements. If the summated cortical electric activity observed in this figure were a "true" visual evoked response, then the response time would be about 150 msec faster than that of the light alone, as determined in the earlier experiments. It would thus appear obvious that, although a time locked phenomenon is observed with the visual stimulus, it is nevertheless different. The probable significance will be discussed later, following the presentation of other cases to show the consistency of these data.

Figure 7 was obtained from another individual. As noted this tracing was

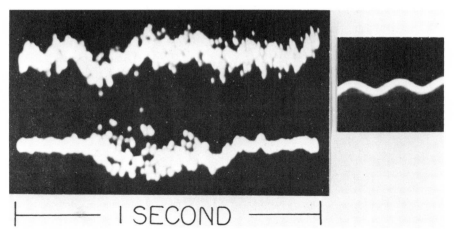

FIG. 6. *Upper line,* cortical evoked responses (CER). *Lower line,* microphone response (MR). Calibration 50 microvolts (RMS), 200X. Positive deflection up in all records.

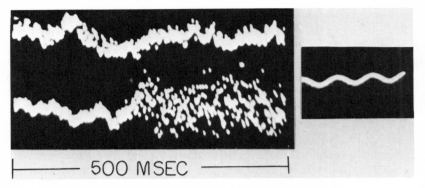

FIG. 7. CER and MR in another patient. 500 msec sweep.

obtained with a more rapid time base (more highly resolved). The first inflection occurred at approximately 60 msec; the peak occurred at 200 msec; the time from the first inflection of the cortical summated activity to the onset of the microphone response was approximately 150 msec.

Figure 8 is shown to demonstrate the general consistency of response in repeated recordings in a given subject. In each instance the first inflection was between 100 and 120 msec, and the time from the first inflection to the micro-. phone rise-front was again in the order of magnitude of approximately 150 msec.

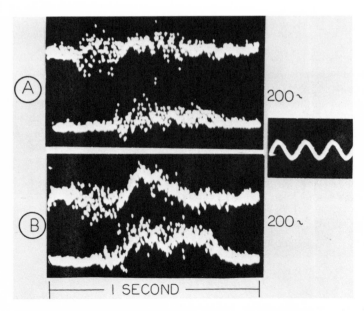

FIG. 8. CER and MR. To show reproducibility in repetitive responses.

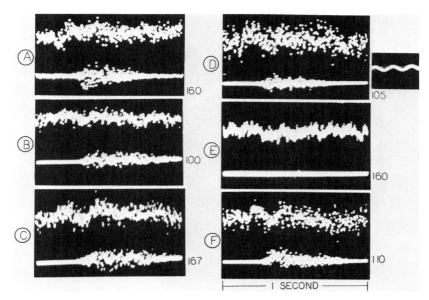

FIG. 9. CER and MR. Repetitive responses. *B* and *C* show build-up of potentials. *E* shows response without phonetic correlates. (See text.)

Figure 9*A* shows the response to the light stimulus of the summated cortical activity, which is again approximately 120 msec for the first inflection and 150 msec for the initiation of the summated microphone response. *B* and *C* of the figure show the build-up of the summated cortical response to light-triggered potentials. *D* again shows the major response in a subsequent series. *E* is the summated cortical potentials when the subject looks at the successive light stimuli but does *not* phonate. In these experiments the subject was told to ignore the numbers completely, but nearly all stated that they could hardly refrain from reading the numbers, primarily because of the afterimagery. In this tracing *E*, some deflection does appear that is time related to the visual triggering, but this is almost insignificant when compared with the subsequent response of *F* with a phonetic output.

For comparison purposes, Fig. 10 was recorded to show the direct electroretinogram and visual evoked response in a normal subject with electrodes placed in the occipital region and the periorbital structures on the same side. An intense light source was used. The initial responses showed a latency of approximately 25 to 30 msec.

DISCUSSION

Using the visual apparatus as input and the initial rise time of phonetic output as the endpoint, two average measurement times were observed: (a) approxi-

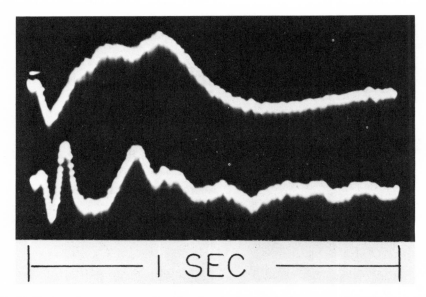

FIG. 10. Electroretinogram, *upper line.* Visual evoked summated response, *lower line,* in normal. To contrast with the evoked response from Broca's area.

mately 500 msec for symbol recognition; and (b) 300 msec for the recognition of "light." The difference obtained in both was considered to be the brain processing time for numeric symbols. This represents the time required to relate the coded visual input pattern to the coded memory for comparison purposes, time to establish the significance of these data for proper set response, retrieval of these data, and then formulation of speech for proper syntax by means of a demultiplexing action and subsequent transmission to Broca's area for the complex motor action of speech. It is obvious that "simple" light recognition also requires complex processing as determined by the long average response time (300 msec). These data are demonstrated in Fig. 11.

From Figs. 6, 7, 8, and 9, it is clear that the orders of magnitudes of the phonetic responses are similar in both the interval timer measurements and the microphone responses in repetitive visual stimulation. The time differences observed appear entirely compatible with the mode of presentation and the set dependent responses.

The summated evoked cortical response that preceded the phonetic action, although related to the visual system activity, is probably not a "true" visual evoked response, but probably represents a command function related to visual activity. These peak times appear roughly time related to elements of the contingent negative variation (CNV) and other stimulus evaluation processes (3,8). Because of the relatively fixed time between the initiation of the phonetic action and the CNV it appears that the latter is indeed a command response; the fixity

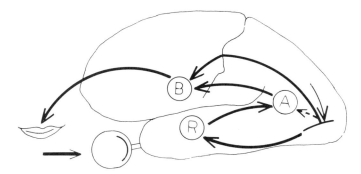

FIG. 11. Diagram of areas corresponding to measurements. R = relating system. A = speech formulation area. B = Broca's area.

of this relationship seems so important that a specific investigation of this detail has been instituted. This command idea is entirely consistent with the work of Mountcastle in which certain parietal lobe units operating from the visual triggering apparatus only fire if the action takes place (6).

The presence of evoked responses to visually triggered potentials over most of the head may be explained as the result of electric spread in an inhomogeneous volume conductor, but the idea is entertained that the scattered responses represent a rough holographic pattern of transfer functions, and that in certain regions of the brain these potentials are, in fact, command and organizing correlates for a given visual input array.

CONCLUSIONS

It has been shown that the normal average subject requires approximately 500 msec to recognize and phonetically produce single digit numerical signals (T_S).

It requires approximately 300 msec using the same system to recognize and respond to a nonsymbol light stimulus (T_L).

Processing time for numeric symbols is defined as $T_S - T_L$, which is approximately 200 msec.

Subjects with disturbed brain function require, on the average, twice the processing time of normals.

In hemi-inattention conditions, the symbol recognition and naming times are at least twofold greater than in the normal side, even with prolonged stimulus times.

Using a summated evoked cortical technique, with electrodes over the orthogonal projection of Broca's area, the data suggest that Broca's area receives command operations from the visual system to activate the complex speech mechanisms.

REFERENCES

1. Cohn, R. (1974): A physiological study of rostral dominance in simultaneously applied ipsilateral somatosensory stimuli. *Mt. Sinai J. Med.,* 41:76–81.
2. Cohn, R. (1975): A physiological model for homologous displacement with paired rostral–caudal stimuli. *Electroencephalogr. Clin. Neurophysiol.,* 38:543.
3. Donchin, E. (1975): On evoked potentials, cognition, and memory. *Science,* 190:1004–1005.
4. Efron, R. (1963): The effect of handedness on the perception of simultaneity and temporal order. *Brain,* 86:261–284.
5. Evarts, E. V. (1974): Sensory motor cortex activity associated with movements triggered by visual as compared to somesthetic inputs. Neuroscience, Third Study Program, edited by Schmitt and Worden. The MIT Press, Cambridge, Massachusetts.
6. Mountcastle, V. B. (1976): The parietal lobe and vision. Eye Institute Seminar, NIH, January 13, 1976.
7. Poffenberger, A. T. (1912): Reaction time to retinal stimulation. *Arch. Psychol.,* 23:1912.
8. Simson, R., Vaughan, H. G., Jr., and Ritter, W. (1976): The scalp topography of potentials associated with missing visual and auditory stimuli. *Electroencephalogr. Clin. Neurophysiol.,* 40: 33–58.

DISCUSSION

Dr. Joynt: In one diagram that you showed with the derivations into the CAT, you had Broca's area on the right side.

Dr. Cohn: This was inadvertently done to direct the face toward the microphone in the diagram. Broca's area, of course, is predominantly located in the left brain.

Dr. Bender: I am sure that you are aware that the rest of the brain participates in occipital lobe and Broca's area interaction; in other words, areas other than those depicted monitor what is expressed. I know you did mention such interaction by the term "mental state." If the mental functions were very much reduced, the values you presented might be quite different.

Dr. Cohn: If the subjects are sick there obviously is a longer duration response time, as noted in my presented data. Furthermore the subject's response time to the light stimulus is not "simple," as is the response to a high intensity stroboscopic flash; this is evident by the much longer latency of verbal response to the numeric light stimulus. As Dr. Bender points out there is a great deal of intracerebral interrelationship. I did not attempt to complicate the diagram by even showing the frontal and parietal components of the response. Recently I heard a very elegant presentation of the role of parietal lobe function in visual mediated responses in the monkey by Mountcastle at NIH in one of Dr. Cogan's seminars. Mountcastle showed that there were time-locked data to the visual stimulus in the parietal lobe; but these units fired only if the animal carried out the act dictated by the visual stimulus. The parietal lobe units thus acted as a sort of command, or consummation, signal. The complexity of visually mediated tasks is likewise shown by the work of Evarts in a recent volume of *Neuroscience.* He showed that if the monkey activated a lever due to a stimulus in the somesthetic cortex there was only a 5 msec delay in the pyramidal tract response. If the monkey had to respond with motor action to visually applied data, it required 100 msec for a response to occur in the pyramidal tract. All these data, including my own, indicate that a tremendous number of cortical interactions are operational to establish proper relations to allow purposeful motor actions. Thus in my work a 300 msec delayed verbal response to "just light" must represent a significantly complex interaction with many complexly organized regions of the brain.

Dr. Bodis-Wollner: When you do the pickup over Broca's area do you have a control of the summated output over the other side?

Dr. Cohn: No.

Dr. Bodis-Wollner: Then doesn't it prejudice your diagram, which was strictly confined to the left side? Wouldn't you be able to make a more complicated (and more precise) diagram of a corpus callosum transfer if you could say that in the control you picked up some similar time locked activity?

Dr. Cohn: Yes, in fact this might result in an exciting series of recordings. It might be that cerebral dominance for motor speech could be elicited by such measurements. This would be particularly true if greater amplitude of output were uniformly observed over the left side in many subjects. From general experience with recording from symmetrical regions of the head I would anticipate that *almost* synchronous potentials would be seen over the homologous brain regions and that the amplitude differences would be significant.

Dr. Bodis-Wollner: When you were talking about the CNV, what exactly was your trigger to the CAT with respect to the red light? I didn't get that.

Dr. Cohn: Only the numeric light signals triggered the response times. The red light that was applied approximately 100 msec prior to the numeric symbol was used to force the subject to look into the midline so as not to prejudice his primary gaze to either side.

Dr. Bodis-Wollner: Well, maybe our understanding of CNV is somewhat different. What did you mean by your use of the term CNV?

Dr. Cohn: The sequences of light stimuli generated an anticipatory response. The subjects knew that the light was to recur at varying intervals, consequently the stimuli were expected. These conditions are therefore basically similar to that employed in any CNV situation.

Dr. Gianbattista: Were the stimulus durations and timing sequences established by electronic means?

Dr. Cohn: No. I am in the process of making such precision measurements. I do not believe that the basic results will be altered significantly.

Dr. Friedland: Were there significantly (or consistently) shorter response times when the light stimulus was applied to either eye?

Dr. Cohn: Statistically no significant lateralization effects were disclosed.

Advances in Neurology, Vol. 18, edited by E. A.
Weinstein and R. P. Friedland. Raven Press,
New York © 1977.

Ocular Movements in Split-Brain Monkeys

Pedro Pasik and Tauba Pasik

*Department of Neurology, Mount Sinai School of Medicine of The City University of
New York, New York, New York 10029*

Many of the presentations in this volume are related to work with so-called
split-brain subjects, and so we selected to present an account of experimental
findings in the monkey, inasmuch as they showed subtle but significant alterations
in oculomotor responses after the section of brain commissures. These disturbances in eye movements can be summarized at the start by stating that disconnection of the hemispheres causes a lateralizing effect or directional preponderance
that becomes evident when split-brain animals are stimulated monocularly. These
effects are present, not only when the movements are elicited in the horizontal
plane, but also in vertical eye deviations.

Eye movements share with all other motor activities of the organism the
characteristic of being evoked by a variety of stimuli. They are, however, exquisitely elicited by visual stimulation. If we restrict ourselves to the latter kind of
ocular deviations, two types have been traditionally recognized, namely the saccade and the smooth pursuit movement (17). Nystagmus can be considered as
a third type, which is distinct from the other two. The saccade is a very rapid
eye movement that occurs in response to a change in the position of the object
of regard. In other words, a saccade is executed when the gaze shifts from one
spot to another spot of the visual field. The stimulus for a smooth pursuit movement is the velocity of the retinal image. This implies that the retinal image must
be in motion. Such motion can be the result of displacement of the stimulus across
the visual field, or it can be produced by movement of the head while fixating
a target. Finally, nystagmus is elicited either by repetitive stimuli traversing the
visual field (optokinetic nystagmus), or it can also be evoked by a stationary
flickering light under certain conditions (flicker-induced nystagmus) (6,8,16).
Both optokinetic nystagmus and flicker-induced nystagmus consist of alternating
rapid and slow phases. The direction of the nystagmus is named by the direction
of the fast phase. It should be noted that fast phases are similar to saccades, and
slow phases resemble smooth pursuit movements. However, as it will be shown
below, it serves no purpose to dissociate the two components of the nystagmic
unit since alterations of nystagmus in a certain direction are usually accompanied
by disturbances of both saccades and smooth pursuit movements in the same
direction.

It has long been known that all of the visually evoked eye movements (saccades, smooth pursuit, and nystagmus), utilize the same functional pathways within the central nervous system. We will review very briefly these pathways, as they were outlined by stimulation and ablation experiments at Mount Sinai during the past almost 40 years (2,7,19). Figure 1 is a diagram of various levels of the monkey brain representing the pathways for conjugate gaze to the right. As indicated, these eye movements are widely represented over the left cerebral hemisphere, mostly in the back and in the front, but on considerably greater areas than the classically delineated occipital and frontal eyefields. These pathways descend in a converging fashion toward the subthalamic region and the midbrain tegmentum. They approach the midline and cross over to the right at the level of the III and IV nerve nuclei in an area ventral to these structures and to the medial longitudinal fasciculus. The pathways become more concentrated close to the midline and descend in the pontine tegmentum between the level of the decussation and the level of the VI nerve nucleus. In this latter region, part of the pathways would presumably activate the right VI nerve nucleus, which will abduct the right eye. The remainder would recross to the left side, ascend through

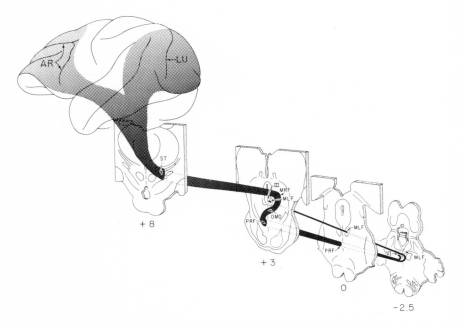

Fig. 1. Diagram of oculomotor pathways as outlined by stimulation and ablation experiments. The cerebral surface and the brain sections are drawn to different scales. AR, arcuate sulcus of frontal lobe; LU, lunate sulcus separating occipital from parietal and temporal lobes; ST, subthalamic region; MRF, mesencephalic reticular formation; III, oculomotor nerve nucleus; OMD, oculomotor decussation; PRF, pontine reticular formation; VI, abducens nerve nucleus; MLF, medial longitudinal fasciculus. Numbers below sections represent anteroposterior stereotaxic coordinates. The graded stippling indicates the location of physiologic pathways for conjugate gaze to the right. (From ref. 14.)

the left medial longitudinal fasciculus, and activate the portion of the left III nerve nucleus innervating the left medial rectus, which will adduct the left eye, thereby completing the conjugate gaze to the right. In fact, anatomic and physiologic evidence suggests that in the area of the VI nerve nucleus there are neurons projecting to the contralateral III nerve nucleus (3,5). Lesions of the oculomotor system result in disturbances of all types of eye movements, namely saccades, smooth pursuit, and nystagmus, to the opposite side when above the decussation and to the same side when below the decussation. Destruction of the medial longitudinal fasciculus interferes with adduction of the ipsilateral eye on attempted gaze to the opposite side. The severity of the oculomotor deficits depends on the size and position of the damage. A large lesion at the level of the cortex, for instance a complete hemidecortication, will interfere severely with all eye movements to the opposite side (9). Similarly, small lesions at the level of the pontine tegmentum will interfere with all eye movements to the ipsilateral side (2). In addition, there is a difference in the relative effect of brain damage on each type of eye movement described above. It is known that defects in optokinetic nystagmus considerably outlast the coexisting deficits in conjugate gaze, as can be seen during the relative recovery of function that occurs after the lesion. Moreover, when the damage is of lesser extent, the disturbances in eye movements may only be revealed by testing for optokinetic nystagmus, since spontaneous saccades and pursuit movements may be within normal limits.

Contrary to the oculomotor pathways that, as outlined above, have been delineated mostly by physiologic methods, the visual pathways have been classically traced with anatomic techniques. It is not necessary to review here the neurohistologic data but for the purposes of this presentation it is important to emphasize that: (a) all optic fibers terminate in various brain structures located rostral to the oculomotor decussation; (b) with the exception of 1 to 2° at the vertical meridian, the representation of the visual fields is exclusively crossed so that input from one side reaches the opposite cerebral hemisphere. It follows from the crossed pattern of the visual and oculomotor systems that an adequate visual stimulus must reach a given side of the brain in order to elicit a normal oculomotor response to the opposite side.

With the preceding background in mind, let us review what happens to visually induced oculomotor phenomena in split-brain monkeys. First of all, spontaneous saccades and smooth pursuit movements are not particularly altered after section of the forebrain commissures. Only when the posterior commissure is severed, the marked disturbances characteristic of the pretectal syndrome become apparent with selective involvement of vertical eye movements (10,14). Examination of optokinetic nystagmus, however, reveals alterations even when the sections are limited to the forebrain. We shall therefore concentrate on the description of this phenomenon.

The general setup for recording optokinetic nystagmus (OKN) is depicted in Fig. 2. A specially designed 35 mm filmloop projector is used to produce four luminous stripes on a rear projection screen. The projected stripes move at a

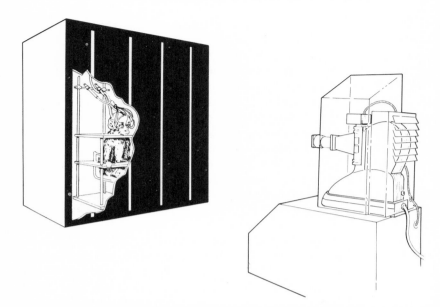

Fig. 2. Set-up for optokinetic stimulation in the horizontal plane. The monkey sits partially restrained behind a rear projection screen on which four luminous stripes are projected. The stripes are 2.5 cm wide and 104 cm long, and are separated by 27.5 cm dark intervals. The luminance of the stripes is 3.5 ftL[1] with 0.99 contrast.

constant speed by way of a servomotor coupled to the film transport mechanism. The monkey is partially restrained in a primate chair with the head relatively fixed. Figure 3 illustrates the electrooculograms of OKN from a normal animal. An important feature brought up by these recordings is that stimulation of only one eye elicits the same response to either side. This is a characteristic of primates, monkeys, and men alike (8). In lower animals that have most of their visual pathways crossing at the optic chiasm, OKN is clearly directional. For example, stimulation of the left eye in the rabbit, which results in classic visual input going mostly to the contralateral cerebral hemisphere, elicits a strong OKN to the left and a weak or absent response to the right (4). In subprimates, therefore, there is a definite lateralizing response in the intact animal.

The first stage in the preparation of a split-brain monkey is the midsagittal section of the optic chiasm as shown in the specimen of Fig. 4a. In such an animal, each eye provides classic visual input only to the ipsilateral side of the brain. According to the previous discussion on the oculomotor pathways, the split of the optic chiasm would create conditions for OKN unidirectionality, i.e., stimulation of the left eye with visual input exclusively directed into the left hemisphere would elicit a good OKN to the right and a poor or absent response to the left. However, the optic chiasm section has no effect on OKN even when stimulation

---

[1] ftL, foot Lambert (unit of luminance).

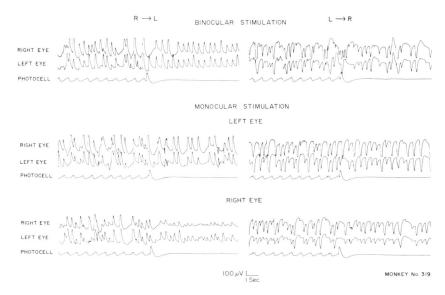

Fig. 3. Electrooculogram of horizontal optokinetic nystagmus in the normal monkey. AC recordings, time constant 0.1 sec. R→L and L→R indicate movement of the stimuli toward the left and right, respectively. O.D., right eye; O.S., left eye; PH, photocell monitoring the stimulus frequency which is 2 Hz. Rapid eye movements to the right or left indicated by deflections of the tracings upward or downward, respectively. Note the continuation of the response (afternystagmus) after cessation of the stimulus. Responses and after responses are the same under both binocular and monocular conditions. (From ref. 8.)

is delivered monocularly. The electrooculograms can not be distinguished from those of a normal animal. The preceding results indicated to us that in the split-chiasm monkey, the visual input from one eye is not in fact restricted to one hemisphere, since, for example, visual information entering the left eye must in some way reach the right hemisphere to produce a normal response to the left. The possibility that brain commissures carry this type of "elementary" information was tested by sectioning the corpus callosum (Fig. 4a, b, c, d). The surgical procedures on the latter structure performed in all studies reported here included the unavoidable destruction of the hippocampal commissure. The results of the combined chiasm-callosum split are depicted in Fig. 5, which is taken from an earlier study (12). Binocular stimulation elicits normal OKN to the right and to the left, whereas monocular stimulation results in a clear dissociation. For example, stimulation of the left eye, i.e., classic input to left hemisphere, produces normal response to the right, but the nystagmus to the left that should be initiated in the right hemisphere is defective. These findings suggest that a given side of the brain receives a visual input from the opposite side through the commissures, in addition to the classic input through the ipsilateral optic tract. The facts that the defect can be reversed by merely changing the stimulated eye and that binocular stimulation results in a normal response, point to a disturbance in

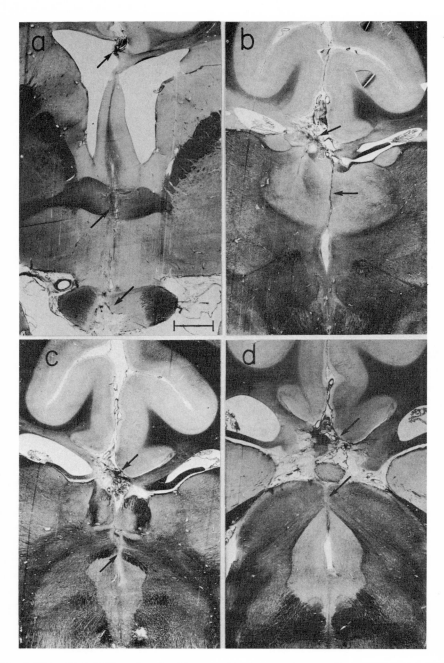

Fig. 4. Midsagittal division of optic chiasm and brain commissures. Representative coronal sections stained for myelin sheaths showing interruption *(arrows)* of the optic chiasm in **a**; corpus callosum in **a, b, c, d**; hippocampal commissure in **b, c, d**; anterior commissure in **a**; massa intermedia in **b**; posterior and habenular commissures in **c**; and intercollicular commissure in **d**. Lesions were made in three stages with intervening testing: optic chiasm; corpus callosum and hippocampal commissure; the remainder forebrain, pretectal and tectal commissures. Note demyelination of crossed optic fibers occupying the core of the chiasm and of the fiber systems crossing the midline. Scale: 2 mm.

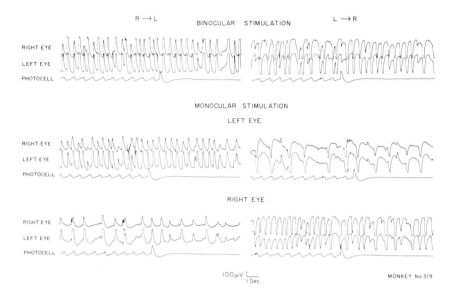

Fig. 5. Electrooculograms of horizontal optokinetic nystagmus after section of optic chiasm and corpus callosum. Notation as in Fig. 3. Note the symmetry of the response to binocular stimulation, and the marked asymmetry under monocular conditions. The deficits appear to the side opposite the "deprived" hemisphere. (From ref. 12.)

input-output integrative processes rather than to a deficit in oculomotor function. Apparently, no adequate visual input is received, for example, by the left cerebral hemisphere on stimulation of the right eye, and, therefore, no appropriate response is made to the right side. Since we have seen already that elimination of the classic visual pathways does not interfere with the response, we are forced to conclude that the additional section of the corpus callosum has produced an interference with visual information that is carried from one to the other side of the brain through this commissure.

The previous experiment was replicated in another preparation in which the optic tract instead of the optic chiasm was sectioned, followed, after intervening testing, by splitting the corpus callosum (13). The section of the right optic tract limits the classic input to the right hemisphere even when binocular stimulation is used. Under these conditions, responses are normal to both sides. Only after the additional section of the corpus callosum, the nystagmus to the left becomes defective, indicating again that commissurotomy abolished an additional visual input to the right cerebral hemisphere. The defective features of the OKN elicited toward the side opposite the visually deprived hemisphere are a marked decrease in the frequency of approximately 50% or more, and the irregular nature of the nystagmic beats, which occur in brief burst and occasionally are difficult to obtain altogether. It should also be noted that in control animals, commissurotomy alone did not produce any deficits.

An important consideration at this point is that in none of the preceding experiments was there a complete abolition of the response. Such results suggest that the so-called deprived hemisphere still receives visual input through some other route. In an attempt to isolate more completely the two hemispheres, the remaining forebrain, pretectal, and tectal commissures, were sectioned in the midline as illustrated in Fig. 4a, b, c, d. The pattern of dysfunction stayed the same, the optokinetic nystagmus opposite to the visually deprived hemisphere was defective, but, despite the extensive disconnection of the telencephalon, diencephalon, pretectal, and tectal regions, there was a failure to completely abolish the response in any direction (13).

We have so far described the oculomotor alterations in split-brain monkeys as revealed by optokinetic stimulation in the horizontal plane. The results indicate that: (a) interfering with the classic visual pathways to one hemisphere, either by monocular stimulation of chiasm-sectioned animals or by simply cutting one optic tract, is not sufficient to totally suppress the visual input to that hemisphere. The remaining input is adequate to initiate the normal optokinetic nystagmus to the opposite side. (b) It appears that both the corpus callosum and some or all of the other forebrain, pretectal, and tectal commissures mediate partially such additional visual inflow. (c) There must be other pathways for the visual input to reach one side of the brain from the contralateral hemisphere, and they may possibly be located in the midbrain tegmentum. Some of our unpublished evidence suggests that input through the accessory optic system could be supplying the visual information necessary for the transfer across the midline at the tegmental level.

The last subject of this presentation concerns the eye movements elicited in the vertical plane. Several lines of evidence have led to the postulation that vertical eye movements are mediated by the same pathways of horizontal gaze to the right and to the left when they are activated simultaneously and bilaterally (1). A typical example in the normal monkey is given by the results of vestibular stimulation. When both ears are simultaneously irrigated with cold water, and the animal is in the erect position, there will ensue a brisk nystagmus in the straight upward direction. Warm water irrigation elicits a nystagmus straight downward. Almost 20 years ago we made these bilateral simultaneous caloric tests on a monkey from which we had previously ablated the cortex of the entire left cerebral hemisphere. The nystagmus obtained was no longer in the strict vertical plane. It had an oblique component toward the side of the hemidecortication (9). A unilateral lesion created an imbalance between the two sides of the brain that prevented the development of the normal pattern of eye movements in the vertical plane. It is important to note that these disturbances consisted of an alteration in the direction and not a total lack of reaction. In other words, the response was still present, but it was oblique instead of vertical. It appeared possible that, similar to the vestibular system, the visual system may also have to be activated bilaterally in order to elicit a normal pattern of vertical ocular deviations. The split-brain preparation is ideal to test this hypothesis. Optokinetic nystagmus in the vertical plane is evoked in the same testing situation of Fig. 1, except that by rotating the filmloop transport mechanism 90°, the projected stripes are horizontal and moved upward or downward with respect to the animal. In the normal monkey, these stimuli produce OKN straight downward or upward, respectively. Vertical optokinetic responses remain unaltered after section of one optic tract or when elicited by monocular stimulation in chiasm-sectioned monkeys, in spite of the fact that under these conditions classic visual input does not reach one of the hemispheres. Such findings suggested again that the so-called deprived hemisphere may receive adequate visual information from the contralateral side through the commissural systems. This hypothesis was, in fact, supported by the findings after additional section of the corpus callosum (11). Figure 6 depicts the electrooculograms obtained from a monkey that had the optic chiasm and the corpus callosum sectioned in the midline. Eye movements are recorded in four channels, one horizontal and one vertical electrode derivation for each eye. This arrangement allows the definition of the direction of eye movements with a good degree of certainty by examining the simultaneous

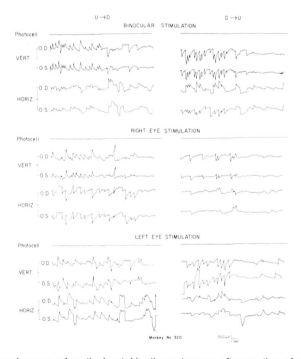

Fig. 6. Electrooculograms of vertical optokinetic nystagmus after section of optic chiasm and corpus callosum. U→D and D→U indicate movement of the stimuli downward and upward, respectively. Other notations as in Fig. 3. Nystagmus is in the strict vertical plane on binocular stimulation. On monocular stimulation, nystagmus is of lower frequency, with an oblique component to the side of the visually "deprived" hemisphere. For recognition of strict vertical and of oblique eye movements see text. (From ref. 11.)

deflections that occur in the four channels. A straight upward movement produces upward deflections in the vertical channels and converging deflections in the horizontal channels. A pure downward movement elicits downward deflections in the vertical channels and divergent deflections in the horizontal channels. When the movement is oblique, for example, upward and to the right, there are upward deflections both in the vertical channels and in the horizontal channels. The method, therefore, permits the recognition of strict vertical eye movements and those with various degrees of obliquity. It is apparent from the recordings of Fig. 6 that binocular stimulation, as expected from bilateral activation, elicits a normal vertical OKN in both upward and downward directions. Contrariwise, monocular stimulation results in abnormal responses of lower frequency and oblique direction. Stripes moving downward elicit a nystagmus upward and to the left when the right eye is open, and upward and to the right when the left eye is stimulated. Similarly, stripes moving upward evoke a downward nystagmus with an oblique component toward the opposite side of the stimulated hemisphere. The same pattern of alterations is observed after section of one optic tract and the corpus callosum. In this case, binocular stimulation is sufficient to reveal the deficits. These results indicate that when visual input is restricted to one hemisphere through interruption of both the classic pathways and the corpus callosum, a normal optokinetic nystagmus in the vertical plane can no longer be elicited. It appears, therefore, that a normal vertical optokinetic nystagmus depends on the bilateral activation of the brain by adequate visual input to both hemispheres.

Taken together, the results of the preceding investigations support the view that "elementary" visual information is carried by brain commissures from one to the other hemisphere. It should be recalled that OKN does not involve learning processes. The phenomenon is present at birth and it does not improve or decay (habituate) with repeated exposures. The findings, therefore, raise questions concerning the transmission of so-called memory traces as the only explanation for the failure of interhemispheric transfer of learning. Moreover, the possible effects of alterations in visuooculomotor reactions that are present in split-brain monkeys should be taken into consideration when evaluating the results of behavioral testing of these animals. As pointed out some 10 years ago as a result of our findings, deficits in horizontal conjugate gaze may cause the neglect of one half of a horizontally arranged discrimination test given to split-brain monkeys (18). This cautionary note should also be extended to include testing situations with vertically displayed targets.

REFERENCES

1. Bender, M. B. (1960): Comments on the physiology and pathology of eye movements in the vertical plane. *J. Nerv. Ment. Dis.*, 130:456–466.
2. Bender, M. B., and Shanzer, S. (1964): Oculomotor pathways defined by electric stimulation and lesions in the brain-stem of monkey. In: *The Oculomotor System*, edited by M. B. Bender, pp. 81–140. Harper & Row, New York.

3. Carpenter, M. B., and McMasters, R. E. (1963): Disturbances of conjugate horizontal eye movements in the monkey. II. Physiological effects and anatomical degeneration resulting from lesions in the medial longitudinal fasciculus. *Arch. Neurol.,* 8:347–368.
4. Fukuda, T., and Tokita, T. (1957): Über die Beziehung der Richtung der optischen Reize zu den Reflextypen der Augen- und Skelettmuskeln. *Acta Otolaryngol.,* 48:415–424.
5. Highstein, S. M., and Baker, R. (1976): Termination of internuclear neurons of the abducens nuclei on medial rectus motoneurons. *Neurosc. Abstr.,* 2:278.
6. Miller, M., Pasik, T., and Pasik, P. (1977): Effect of visual field homogeneity on flicker-induced nystagmus in monkeys. *Fed. Proc.,* 36:508.
7. Pasik, P., and Pasik, T. (1964): Oculomotor functions in monkeys with lesions of the cerebrum and the superior colliculi. In: *The Oculomotor System,* edited by M. B. Bender, pp. 40–80. Harper & Row, New York.
8. Pasik, P. and Pasik, T. (1975): A comparison between two types of visually-evoked nystagmus in the monkey. *Acta Otolaryngol. Suppl.,* 330:30–37.
9. Pasik, P., Pasik, T., and Bender, M. B. (1960): Oculomotor function following cerebral hemidecortication in the monkey: A study with special reference to optokinetic and vestibular nystagmus. *Arch. Neurol.,* 3:298–305.
10. Pasik, P., Pasik, T., and Bender, M. B. (1969): The pretectal syndrome in monkeys: I. Disturbances of gaze and body posture. *Brain,* 92:521–534.
11. Pasik, P., Pasik, T., Valciukas, J. A., and Bender, M. B. (1971): Vertical optokinetic nystagmus in the split-brain monkey. *Exp. Neurol.,* 30:162–171.
12. Pasik, T., and Pasik, P. (1964): Optokinetic nystagmus: An unlearned response altered by section of chiasm and corpus callosum in monkeys. *Nature,* 203:609–611.
13. Pasik, T., and Pasik, P. (1972): Transmission of "elementary" visual information through brain commissures as revealed by studies on optokinetic nystagmus in monkeys. In: *Cerebral Interhemispheric Relations,* edited by J. Cernacek and F. Podivinsky, pp. 267–285. Publ. House Slovak Acad. Sc., Bratislava.
14. Pasik, T., and Pasik, P. (1975): Experimental models of oculomotor dysfunction in the rhesus monkey. In: *Primate Models of Neurological Disorders,* edited by B. S. Meldrum and C. D. Marsden, pp. 77–89. Raven Press, New York.
15. Pasik, T., Pasik, P., and Bender, M. B. (1969): The pretectal syndrome in monkeys. II. Spontaneous and induced nystagmus and "lightning" eye movements. *Brain,* 92:871–884.
16. Pasik, T., Pasik, P., and Valciukas, J. A. (1970): Nystagmus induced by stationary repetitive light flashes in monkeys. *Brain Res.,* 19:313–317.
17. Rashbass, C. (1961): The relationship between saccadic and smooth tracing eye movements. *J. Physiol.,* 159:326–338.
18. Trevarthen, C. (1964): Functional interactions between the cerebral hemispheres of the split-brain monkey. In: *Functions of the Corpus Callosum,* edited by G. Ettlinger, pp. 24–41. Churchill, London.
19. Wagman, I. H. (1964): Eye movements induced by electric stimulation of cerebrum in monkeys and their relationship to bodily movements. In: *The Oculomotor System,* edited by M. B. Bender, pp. 18–39. Harper & Row, New York.

DISCUSSION

Dr. Bodis-Wollner: Do you think that all information transfer through the posterior corpus callosum involves low level signals, and is some of that information already elaborated by one side of the posterior cortex?

Dr. Pedro Pasik: There is some electrophysiologic information pointing to the fact that there is no need to postulate transmission of "higher level signals" through the corpus callosum. In the late 60s the Italian investigators, Berlucchi and his co-workers (Gazzaniga was in that laboratory at the time) plotted the visual receptive fields from fiber units in the posterior corpus callosum of the cat and found that such receptive fields were indistinguishable from those described as typical of visual cortex neurons. These findings supported our interpretation.

Advances in Neurology, Vol. 18, edited by E. A.
Weinstein and R. P. Friedland. Raven Press,
New York © 1977.

Concluding Remarks

Edwin A. Weinstein and Robert P. Friedland

*Department of Neurology, Mount Sinai Medical School, New York, New York 10029;
and Veterans Administration Hospital, Bronx, New York 10468*

This volume has brought together clinical observations of unilateral neglect, the results of localized lesions in animals, the effects of section of the corpus callosum in man, and data derived from studies of hemisphere interactions in normal human subjects. The major issues were the definition of hemi-neglect and the determination of whether its manifestations should be differentiated from those of sensory extinction; the role of selective and motivational factors; the predominance of left-sided neglect over right-sided hemi-inattention; and their relationship to other aspects of hemisphere specialization.

The various clinical phenomena of hemi-neglect and the methods of examination were reviewed. Extinction and its motor analog, shift of the eyes to the unaffected side on the presentation of paired visual stimuli, were described. As several observers pointed out, this eye shift, originally reported by Cohn, occurs even when both stimuli are placed in the seeing field of a hemianopic subject. The chapters of Bender (Chap. 8) and Weinstein and Friedland (Chap. 4) make a sharp distinction between extinction and the more conspicuous manifestations of hemi-neglect. These authors report that severe neglect is invariably associated with other disturbances of behavior, notably of mood and consciousness, while extinction itself, may be elicited on DSS, in the presence of a relatively normal mental status. Second, they note that extinction is more enduring than the more severe signs of neglect; and third, that there is no lateralized predominance of one side over the other in cases of unimodal extinction. Heilman and Watson (Chap. 7), on the other, do not postulate separate mechanisms, but believe that all the manifestations of unilateral neglect are aspects of a defect in arousal and in the orienting response. Kinsbourne proposes that all the various sensory and visuomotor signs are a result of an alteration in transcallosal inhibitory mechanisms involving different levels of complexity.

Joynt has given us some crucial information on this issue. He notes that the clinical manifestations of hemi-neglect following callosal section in man are inconspicuous. This is contrary to what one would expect if the corpus callosum were regarded as the sole conduit for the transfer of information from one side of the body and/or space to the opposite hemisphere. Dr. Joynt points out that there are other information systems that do not travel across the corpus callosum. This viewpoint is supported by the experimental findings of the Pasiks. They found that extracallosal interhemispheric pathways mediate adequate visual input to elicit normal optokinetic responses in both the horizontal and vertical planes. The right hemisphere does "know" and is "conscious" of a great deal of what is going on, in the left field of space. Like an aphasic patient, it cannot give a specific label but it manifests knowledge in emotional language and gesture. In this sense, the right hemisphere is both conscious and attentive. The preservation of consciousness is in accordance with the intactness of the connections between the two halves of the brain through the brainstem commissures.

As Heilman and Watson have shown, it is these structures and their corticolimbic connections that must be damaged for conspicuous hemi-neglect to occur. One would expect that if, in the operative procedure of severing the great callosal commissure, surrounding structures like the fornix and cingulate area were damaged, then there would be more marked neglect than has been reported by Joynt or noticed by others.

The evidence from callosal section indicates that, in health, the corpus callosum serves the important function of inhibiting extinction and that its section increases the imbalance between the hemispheres, accentuating the types of extinction and completion that were so strikingly demonstrated by Levy. In contrast, the patient with marked hemi-neglect does not simply blot out one side, but conceptualizes the affected side as "missing," or belonging to some one else, etc. Cohn provided some significant measurements in his distinction of the mechanisms of input processing and symbolic processing times. In addition, the data presented by the Pasiks emphasized the importance of possible visuo-oculomotor alterations in the evaluation of experimental results in split brain animals.

The mechanisms whereby damage to the limbic-reticular system results in conspicuous hemi-neglect was not made entirely clear. The explanation that the emotional language and dramatic gestures in which the patient represents one side of the body and ambient space is due to loss of cortical control is not borne out by the results of cortical ablation. Following removal of the right parietal cortex by Dr. Wilder Penfield for seizures and painful phantom limbs, Henry Hecaen found contralateral extinction and marked constructional difficulties but relatively little hemi-neglect beyond the immediate postoperative period. Similarly, even after hemispherectomy, there is extinction but not conspicuous hemi-neglect. The explanation offered by Heilman and Watson is that lesions which interrupt cortico-reticular loops produced a unilateral defect in arousal and in the orienting response. Weinstein and Friedland suggest that the limbic lesion converts extinction to more marked hemi-inattention, an effect also produced by drugs such as barbiturates that affect the limbic-reticular system.

The role of motivational and psychological factors was well illustrated by Diller and Weinberg. As was pointed out in the discussion of their chapter, there is a tendency for the conspicuous signs of unilateral neglect to clear spontaneously, but their patients did show impressive behavioral changes, whatever the interpretation. The adaptational and maladaptational features are also shown in the frequent association with verbal denial. Here an ultimate answer awaits the result of further investigations, such as those of Vernon Mountcastle, who has demonstrated that there are mechanisms for the selective registration of events in hemi-space linked to survival functions.

In Chapter 4, the relationship to unilateral neglect of the associated disturbances in mood and consciousness, such as verbal denial, disorientation, reduplications, non-aphasic misnaming and self-referential interpretations of proverbs and idioms was considered. The view was that these are forms of altered metaphor in which the patient conceptualizes his environment in a manner similar to the way he represents the affected hemi-body and hemi-space in confabulations, delusions, personifications, and humour. Weinstein and Friedland also regard some of the non-verbal aspects of unilateral neglect; those other than extinction and eye shift, as forms of gesture in which the affected side is represented. While the patient does not, in referential language, express "conscious" awareness of the hemi-space, he seems to indicate awareness at a less "conscious" level.

Another writer who has addressed the significance of the associated verbal denial and confabulations is Norman Geschwind. Geschwind regards unilateral neglect as the manifestation of a disconnexion of the right parietal lobe from the language centers of the left hemisphere. The confabulation is seen as the compensation for the lack of conscious awareness of the left hemi-space.

Several explanations of the predominance of left over right sided unilateral neglect were offered. Kinsbourne described the natural tendency of man and many other species to orient to the right, and made the point that this is a force that transcends individual sensory and motor modalities. Neglect of the left side is accentuated when the left hemisphere is activated by the verbal thought processes involved in the neurological examination, causing inhibition of the right hemisphere and erasure of the perception of the left side. Heilman approached the problem from the standpoint of possible anatomical and neurotransmitter differences between the hemispheres. It may be that corticofugal pathways were more discretely organized in the right hemisphere so that a localized lesion would damage more units. He also suggested that there might be a difference in dopamine metabolism in the two hemispheres, citing the work of Ungerstedt, who produced hemi-neglect in rats by chemically inactivating the dopaminergic pathway.

The explanation of Weinstein and Friedland for the predominance of left-sided hemi-neglect is based on the difference in linguistic functions of the hemispheres and the paucity of metaphorical speech and gesture with left hemisphere lesions. Because such patients cannot use the colorful metaphor and vivid gesture that characterize severe unilateral neglect and verbal anosognosia, right-sided hemi-inattention is not only less frequent, but less severe than is the case of a right hemisphere lesion. When marked right-sided hemi-neglect does appear, it is commonly associated with jargon aphasia; a combination of a fluent aphasia, verbal denial, and a disturbance of consciousness, in effect an unsuccessful attempt to use metaphorical speech.

These views support the belief of Hughlings Jackson that both hemispheres are involved in speech, with the right hemisphere having a role beyond that of a less skilled substitute, to be called upon only in dire situations. Rather than stating that the left hemisphere is specialized for language and the right hemisphere is dominant for affect, it may be more accurate to say that the left hemisphere is dominant for the phonological, sequential, syntactic, and referential aspects of language and the right is the leading hemisphere for the sensory-ideational and experiential features of language.

Glossary

Term	Reference	Definition
Agnosia for left half of space	Brain (1941)	left hemi-neglect with turning to the right
Algohallucinosis	Van Bogaert, quoted by Critchley (1953)	recurrent episodes of feeling of disappearance of affected side with dizziness and spontaneous pain in paralyzed arm
Akinetic mutism	Cairns, Oldfield, Pennybacker, and Whitteridge (1941)	a condition in which there is a marked paucity of voluntary movement, though the eyes regard the observer steadily and follow objects, in which the patient does not speak or talks in whispered monosyllables, in which he can swallow, but has to be fed, and in which there is no expression of emotion
Allesthesia	Jones (1907) Bender et al. (1948)	displacement of a single stimulus to a homologous site on the other side of the body
Allochiria	Obersteiner (1881)	uncertainty as to which side of body has been touched, also dyschiria
Amnesia for body half	Nielson (1938a) Cobb (1947)	hemi-neglect
Amorphosynthesis	Denny-Brown (1952, 1963)	unilateral distortion of perception resulting in a unilateral disorder of behavior at the physiological level
Anosodiaphoria	Babinski (1914)	lack of concern about hemiparesis
Anosognosia of Babinski	Babinski (1914)	lack of awareness of hemiplegia, literal lack of knowledge of disease
Anosognosie vraie ou muette	Van Bogaert, quoted by Critchley (1953)	asomatognosia, sense of nothingness
Anton's syndrome	Anton (1899)	denial or unawareness of blindness, usually associated with bilateral lesion of visual cortex, but denial or unawareness of blindness may also be seen with lesions of the optic chiasm (eds)

References cited are listed in Chapter 1.

Term	Authors	Description
Apractognosia Aschématie	Grünbaum (1930) Bonnier (1905)	visual constructive derangement diminished awareness of the body, also hyposchematie (hyperschematie—positive sensory features as increased heaviness, sensation of swollen limb)
Autoheterosyncisis Autosomatamnesia	Critchley (1953) Gerstmann (1942)	patient confuses his own limbs with those of examiner "a dissociation from memory . . . with forgetting of the existence or nonrecognition of the possession of defective body parts"
Autosomatognosia	Gerstmann (1942)	also mono- or hemi- "dissociation from conscious recognition of individual defective parts of the entire side of the body"
Autotopagnosia	Pick (1922)	also hemi- and mono- loss of ability for recognition of and orientation to body parts of self and others, without awareness of defect
Confabulation	Weinstein and Lyerly (1968)	a fictitious narrative of some past event or events, a condensed symbolic or metaphorical representation of current problems or relationships, given in the past tense
Constructional apraxia	Kleist (1934)	defective visual control of manual activity
Disorientation for date	Paterson and Zangwill (1944); Weinstein and Kahn (1955)	gross errors in designation of month and/or year
Disorientation for place	Paterson and Zangwill (1944), Weinstein and Kahn (1955)	misdesignation and erroneous location of where the patient is—includes misnaming, mislocation, condensation of distance between home and hospital, and confabulated journey
Disorientation for time of day	Weinstein and Kahn (1955)	errors in designation of time, with confusing of A.M. and P.M.; morning, afternoon, and evening

Term	Author(s)	Description
Displacement	Bender (1952)	incorrect localization on the body of one of two simultaneously applied stimuli
Double stimulation (doppelte Erriezung)	Oppenheim (1885)	method of sensory testing using two simultaneously applied stimuli
Exosomesthesia	Shapiro, Fink and Bender (1952)	displacement of cutaneous sensation into extra personal space on **DSS**
Extinction	Bender (1952)	"a process in which a sensation disappears or becomes imperceptible when another sensation is evoked by simultaneous stimulation elsewhere in the sensory field"
Hemianopic weakness of attention	Poppelreuter (1917)	visual extinction
Hemianopsie relative	Thiebault and Guillaumet	visual extinction
Hemiasomatognosia	Critchley (1953)	feeling of nothingness or unawareness of one half of the body
Hemidepersonalization	Ehrenwald (1930)	loss of awareness of one body half
Identification anosognosia	Critchley (1953)	sensation that limbs of one side are missing and are replaced by those of another person
Illusions of corporeal transformation and displacement	Hecaen and Ajuriaguerra (1952)	sensation of affected body part becoming swollen, elongated, and separated from body
Imperception	Jackson (1876)	lack of recognition of objects, persons, and places
Imperception	Denny-Brown (1952)	"inability to reach a conclusion regarding the origin of multiple sensory data, the primary data being intact"
Imperception for one half of body	Schilder and Critchley (1953)	feeling of nothingness of one half of the body

Term	Reference	Definition
Jargon aphasia	Weinstein, Kahn, Lyerly and Ozer (1966) Kinsbourne and Warrington (1963)	a form of fluent aphasia in which large portions of the patient's speech are not comprehensible to auditors, while the patient himself is unaware of, or denies a speech disturbance; speech may contain neologisms or standard English words used in an apparently meaningless context
Local adaptation	P. Cibis and Müller (1948)	tactile extinction
Ludic behavior	Weinstein, Kahn, and Sugarman (1954)	a term initially used by Jean Piaget to describe the play, imitative, and dramatic aspects of the behavior of young children
Misoplegia	Critchley (1974)	hatred of hemiplegia
Motor impersistence	Fisher (1956)	the inability to sustain a movement that has been initiated on command
Nonaphasic misnaming	Weinstein and Kahn (1952)	the selective misnaming of objects connected with illness or some other personal problem or relationship
Obscuration	Bender (1952)	diminished intensity of a perception on DSS
Optic apraxia	Kleist (1912)	apraxic disturbance of drawing with misdirected grasping and pointing
Organic repression	Schilder (1935)	excluding unpleasant features of illness from consciousness in patients with organic brain disease, a process similar to psychic repression, but due to organic factors
Pain asymbolia	Schilder and Stengel (1928)	absence of the normal reactions to noxious stimuli as a result of acquired cerebral lesions with intact elementary sensation
Pain hemiagnosia	Hecaen (1962)	nonrecognition on one half of the body of the nature and place of painful stimuli, which are felt nonetheless

Term	Reference	Description
Painful anosognosia	Van Bogaert (1934)	spontaneous pains and postural distortion in affected limbs
Personification anosognosia	Juba (1949)	organic paranoid reaction with possession of paralyzed limb being referred to someone else
Personification of the paralyzed limbs	Critchley (1955)	regarding of paralyzed extremities as a foreign body, as if they had a personal identity all their own
Planotopokinesia	Marie, Bouttier, and Baily (1922)	loss of conception of topographical relationships
Pseudohemianopia	Silberpfennig (1941)	inability to respond to visual stimuli in one homonymous field contralateral to frontal lobe lesion
Pseudomoria	Babenkova (1976)	euphoria, excessive familiarity, loss of tact, excessive joking, and discussion of sexuality with unawareness of illness and confabulation seen with right posterior hemisphere lesions
Pseudopolymelia	Kanareikin et al. (1976)	feeling of third hand or foot (reduplication of body parts)
Psychic hemiplegia	Fisher (1956)	failure to use a limb in gesture in the absence of significant motor or sensory deficit
Reduplication for body parts	Weinstein and Kahn (1955)	the statement that one has an additional body part, such as another left or right arm or multiple heads
Reduplication for person	Weinstein, Kahn, and Sugarman (1952)	the statement that a person has more than one identity with the same or similar name, such as the belief that a doctor is also an insurance agent
Reduplication for place	Weinstein, Kahn, and Sugarman (1952)	the fictitious statement that there are two or more places (usually the hospital) of the same or similar names, whereas only one exists in reality
Reduplication for time	Weinstein, Kahn, and Sugarman (1952)	the fictitious statement that a current experience has also occurred in the past; an enduring déjà vu experience

Term	Reference	Description
Reduplicative paramnesia	Pick (1903)	the erroneous belief that an actual current experience is a duplication of a previous one
Segmental depersonalization	Ehrenwald (1931)	unacceptance or even denial of one's own excreta or products of menstruation
Sensory eclipse	G. Vercelli (1947)	extinction
Sensory suppression	Reider (1946) Furmanski (1950)	extinction
Somatognosia (hemisomatognosia)	Hecaen (1962)	body scheme disturbance, ranging from complete unawareness of one body half to unilateral finger agnosia
Somatoparaphrenia	Gerstmann (1942)	specific psychic elaboration with illusional, confabulatory, or delusional ideas in reference to experience of absence of the affected limbs or side of body
Somatotopagnosia	Gerstmann (1942)	"a primary disturbance or loss of ability for recognition of and orientation as to the various parts of the body (one's own as well as that of others) and their spatial interrelation", without awareness by the patient
Supernumerary phantom	Critchley (1953) Jones (1907)	feeling of third arm or leg; reduplication of body parts
Synchiria		touch on one hand referred to both sides
Synesthesia	Bender (1952)	when a single stimulus evokes two sensations, one at the point of stimulation and another in a different region, "usually displaced toward an area of the body which is spontaneously painful or shows dysesthesia; an area which is charged with a great deal of emotional tone"
Tactile inattention	Critchley (1949)	tactile extinction
Tactile ineffectiveness	Goldstein (1949)	tactile extinction
Unilateral spatial agnosia	Duke Elder (1949)	unawareness of the left half of space

Visual disorientation	Holmes (1919)	defective object localization
Visual inattention	Holmes (1919)	limitation of visual attention to objects in central vision
Visual inattention	Poppelreuter (1917)	visual extinction
Visuospatial agnosia	Paterson and Zangwill (1944)	defective analysis of spatial relationships in execution of constructional tasks under visual control

Index